3rd Edition

Communication & Interpersonal Skills in Nursing

Shirley Bach & Alec Grant

Los Angeles | London | New Delhi
Singapore | Washington DC | Boston

Learning Matters
An imprint of SAGE Publications Ltd
1 Oliver's Yard
55 City Road
London EC1Y 1SP

SAGE Publications Inc.
2455 Teller Road
Thousand Oaks, California 91320

SAGE Publications India Pvt Ltd
B 1/I 1 Mohan Cooperative Industrial Area
Mathura Road
New Delhi 110 044

SAGE Publications Asia-Pacific Pte Ltd
3 Church Street
#10-04 Samsung Hub
Singapore 049483

Editor: Alex Clabburn
Development editor: Richenda Milton-Daws
Production controller: Chris Marke
Project management: Swales & Willis Ltd,
Exeter, Devon
Marketing manager: Camille Richmond
Cover design: Wendy Scott
Typeset by: C&M Digitals (P) Ltd, Chennai, India
Printed by CPI Group (UK) Ltd, Croydon, CR0 4YY

First edition published 2009 by Learning Matters Ltd
Second edition published 2011
Third edition published 2015

Library of Congress Control Number: 2014956109

British Library Cataloguing in Publication data

A catalogue record for this book is available from the British Library

MIX
Paper from
responsible sources
FSC
www.fsc.org   FSC® C013604

ISBN 978-1-4739-0256-5
ISBN 978-1-4739-0257-2 (pbk)

Contents

Transforming Nursing Practice is a series tailor-made for pre-registration student nurses. Each book in the series is:

- ○ Affordable
- ○ Mapped to the NMC Standards and Essential Skills Clusters
- ○ Full of active learning features
- ○ Focused on applying theory to practice

Each book addresses a core topic and they have been carefully developed to be simple to use, quick to read and written in clear language.

> "
> An invaluable series of books that explicitly relates to the NMC standards.
> Each book cover a different topic that students need to explore in order
> to develop into a qualified nurse… I would recommend this series to all
> Pre-Registration nursing students whatever their field or year of study
>
> **Linda Robson**
> **Senior Lecturer, Edge Hill University**
>
> The set of books is an excellent resource for students. The series is small,
> easily portable and valuable. I use the whole set on a regular basis.
>
> **Fiona Davies**
> **Senior Nurse Lecturer, University of Derby**
>
> I recommend the SAGE/Learning Matters series to all my students
> as they are relevant and concise. Please keep up the good work.
>
> **Thomas Beary**
> **Senior Lecturer in Mental Health Nursing, University of Hertfordshire**
> "

ABOUT THE SERIES EDITORS

Professor Shirley Bach is Head of the School of Health Sciences at the University of Brighton and responsible for the core knowledge titles. Previously she was head of post-graduate studies and has developed curriculum for undergraduate and pre-registration courses in a variety of subject domains.

Dr Mooi Standing is an Independent Academic Consultant (UK and International) and responsible for the personal and professional learning skills titles. She is an accredited NMC Quality Assurance Reviewer of educational programmes and a Professional Regulator Panellist on the NMC Practice Committee.

Sandra Walker is Senior Teaching Fellow in Mental Health at the University of Southampton and responsible for the mental health nursing titles. She is a Qualified Mental Health Nurse with a wide range of clinical experience spanning more than 20 years.

CORE KNOWLEDGE TITLES:

Becoming a Registered Nurse: Making the Transition to Practice
Communication and Interpersonal Skills in Nursing (3rd Ed)
Contexts of Contemporary Nursing (2nd Ed)
Getting into Nursing (2nd Ed)
Health Promotion and Public Health for Nursing Students (2nd Ed)
Introduction to Medicines Management in Nursing
Law and Professional Issues in Nursing (3rd Ed)
Leadership, Management and Team Working in Nursing (2nd Ed)
Learning Skills for Nursing Students
Medicines Management in Children's Nursing
Nursing and Collaborative Practice (2nd Ed)
Nursing and Mental Health Care
Nursing in Partnership with Patients and Carers
Passing Calculations Tests for Nursing Students (3rd Ed)
Palliative and End of Life Care in Nursing
Patient Assessment and Care Planning in Nursing (2nd Ed)
Patient and Carer Participation in Nursing
Patient Safety and Managing Risk in Nursing
Psychology and Sociology in Nursing (2nd Ed)
Successful Practice Learning for Nursing Students (2nd Ed)
Understanding Ethics in Nursing Practice
Using Health Policy in Nursing
What is Nursing? Exploring Theory and Practice (3rd Ed)

PERSONAL AND PROFESSIONAL LEARNING SKILLS TITLES:

Clinical Judgement and Decision Making for Nursing Students (2nd Ed)
Critical Thinking and Writing for Nursing Students (2nd Ed)
Evidence-based Practice in Nursing (2nd Ed)
Information Skills for Nursing Students
Reflective Practice in Nursing (2nd Ed)
Succeeding in Essays, Exams & OSCEs for Nursing Students
Succeeding in Literature Reviews and Research Project Plans for Nursing Students (2nd Ed)
Successful Professional Portfolios for Nursing Students (2nd Ed)
Understanding Research for Nursing Students (2nd Ed)

MENTAL HEALTH NURSING TITLES:

Assessment and Decision Making in Mental Health Nursing
Engagement and Therapeutic Communication in Mental Health Nursing
Medicines Management in Mental Health Nursing
Mental Health Law in Nursing
Physical Healthcare and Promotion in Mental Health Nursing
Psychosocial Interventions in Mental Health Nursing

ADULT NURSING TITLES:

Acute and Critical Care in Adult Nursing
Caring for Older People in Nursing
Medicines Management in Adult Nursing
Nursing Adults with Long Term Conditions
Safeguarding Adults in Nursing Practice
Dementia Care in Nursing

You can find more information on each of these titles and our other learning resources at **www.sagepub.co.uk**. Many of these titles are also available in various e-book formats, please visit our website for more information.

Foreword to the first edition

As someone who supports students in clinical placements, I am struck by how often it is that the subtle intricacies around how we communicate and interact with patients, families and colleagues present us as nurses with the greatest intellectual and emotional challenges. Numerous dilemmas, confusions, misunderstandings and anxieties arise as we try to tease out what we bring to the game as individuals, what we encounter in our roles as students and nurses, and what are complex aspects of the patients, relatives, professionals and organisations we engage with.

It is in this light that I welcome this excellent book, in which the authors span a breadth of interesting, pertinent and at times refreshing topics that are important in considering communication and interpersonal skills in all fields of nursing. In places, rather demanding concepts are explored, but it is worth the effort as the authors illuminate nursing practice by drawing on core evidence from nursing and then venture outside the traditional stomping ground to pull in research, theories and ideas belonging to other fields. This lateral approach promises to stimulate nursing students and others to explore how best to make sense of the complexities and challenges of communication and interpersonal relationships.

The book looks at some of the typical stumbling blocks many of us encounter as we strive to learn how to communicate and interact safely and effectively, and offers ways to anticipate and engage with the potential barriers that often lead to emotional struggles for students in practice. Practical can-do exercises within these pages offer students scope to reflect on their personal and clinical experiences and relate these to the focus of a particular chapter. Many of these interactive elements could prove to be prize material in class-based teaching and learning.

The chapter on the learning and educational context should be valuable to many students and mentors as it provides a wholesale exploration of how the student experience, both in university and practice, fits within a broader educational framework. The results of engaging with this should be a more empowered student who takes greater ownership of their education and mentors that can better appreciate how the sum of the parts fits together.

The last two chapters shed a bright light on the social-cultural settings within which nursing practice, interpersonal interactions and communication take place. These rich, thoughtful and wide-ranging sections scrutinise the challenges of providing effective healthcare across the lifespan within a constantly evolving, diverse society.

I came away from reading this book with new concepts and understanding that will inform my work with students and qualified nurses for years to come. It is with great pleasure that I commend it to you.

Dr Alan Simpson

Senior Research Fellow and Lecturer

Vice-Chair, Mental Health Nurse Academics (UK)

City University, London

Foreword to the third edition

The fact that this text is in its third edition is testament not only to the popularity of the book but to the requirement for ongoing information within the nursing profession on this important area of practice. One underpinning theme within this book is the number of ironies associated with healthcare communication. The first of these is highlighted early on. Nursing students entering their programme of study are already experts, as communication is 'learned since birth'. While there is often excitement upon presentation of the range of clinical skills and nursing care topics, lectures, tutorials and small-group teaching of communication skills can be met with a certain reluctance, in so far as many students have been practising these basic skills for at least 17 years and many have already received some instruction on the topic. Thus imparting the basics of communication in a way that engages students can be difficult. Additionally historical and popular rhetoric, emphasised more recently in screening for 'compassion' among potential nursing students, lends credence to the notion that a person has the 'personality' to be a nurse and by default may not need that much input in communication theory and skills.

To this end Bach and Grant clearly challenge nursing students to reconsider communication as a taken-for-granted skill. They do this in part by presenting the second underpinning irony, and that is that healthcare workers generally overestimate their skills in this domain, while at the same time both nationally and internationally communication failings account for the largest proportion of hospital complaints. Similarly, national healthcare failures, such as those outlined in the Francis report (2013), highlight endemic communication lapses in terms of respect and dignity.

This complacency is possibly reinforced by positive feedback (or lack of negative feedback) received from clients during care experiences, as they generally don't complain. Bach and Grant very clearly expose the vulnerability of clients in this regard, developed most strongly in the notion of mental patients as 'survivors' to jolt us as a profession to re-examine our behaviours in this regard. Similarly, this book raises awareness of the need for culturally sensitive communication, without which, unbeknownst to ourselves, we operate from our own cultural lenses.

The final irony is that we have never had it so good. People are generally wealthier and better educated than when the National Health Service began. Nursing has grown as a profession, underpinned by evidence with an abundance of supportive literature (both research and textbooks) to support practice. And yet the very fundamentals of nursing (and human service) of person-centred approach are often missing. The reasons for this are varied, but include the general 'business' that health professionals like to adopt, as Bach and Grant outline, and a focus on tasks that can potentially lead to dehumanising patients in our care.

At the same time Bach and Grant provide an interesting perspective that highlights the burden that nurses sometimes face. Being personally accountable for care and required to reflect and develop effective communication skills can be challenging within some organisations and cultures. Bach and Grant point out that, in some respects, the nurse is powerless to change elements of communication and put it to organisations to take responsibility for and explore environmental factors that undermine good communication.

Bach and Grant confront many of these ironies in a subtle yet clear way. Nursing students are challenged to learn and develop communication skills. The book serves as a useful and easy-to-read resource that provides the necessary content which is reinforced by many student activities, scenarios and exercises. Additional readings and website resources are also very appropriate and useful. Critical reflection and lifelong learning are useful concepts that are explored in the book. These emphasise that the nursing student – rather than expert – is and will always be a learner. Communication skills need continuous reflection and development using personal awareness and reflection and listening to the people that we care for.

This book is an excellent read. It is a must-have for the bookshelf. Including a newly developed chapter and using comprehensive resources, Bach and Grant provide a straightforward, easy-to-read handbook for nursing students and nurses to build and develop communication skills. At the same time there is subtle consciousness raising and challenges to the status quo that are essential in today's healthcare environment.

Dr Fiona Timmins
Associate Professor
School of Nursing and Midwifery
Trinity College Dublin

About the authors

Professor Shirley Bach is Professor of Nursing Education and Head of the School of Health Sciences at the University of Brighton and also the Series Editor for *Transforming Nursing Practice*. In the past, she has designed curricula for nurses that integrated interpersonal relationship skills with communication studies, before specialising in health psychology and the application of psychology to health and illness settings. She has written a study guide in psychology for nurses, and researched and developed a model for psychological care. Shirley has also led programmes that promote the professional practice of nursing and midwifery, especially in the area of advanced nursing practice, and has co-authored another text in the *Transforming Nursing Practice* series on *Leadership, Management and Team Working in Nursing*. More recently, she has developed an interest in new learning technologies and has drawn upon her understanding both of communication and of pedagogic theories to publish in this area.

Dr Alec Grant is Reader in Narrative Mental Health in the School of Health Sciences at the University of Brighton. He qualified as a mental health nurse in the mid-1970s and went on to study psychology, social science and psychotherapy. He is widely published in the fields of ethnography, autoethnography, narrative inquiry, clinical supervision, cognitive behavioural psychotherapy, and communication and interpersonal skills. His current and developing scholarly interests coalesce broadly in the area of narrative research, and postmodern and poststructural developments in qualitative inquiry, in mental health and other healthcare areas.

Acknowledgements

The authors and publisher would like to thank the following University of Brighton students: Kate Morris, for making such helpful suggestions for revisions to the first edition of this book, and Amy Barlow and Jaime Naish for their equivalent contributions to this edition. We would also like to thank Dr Helen Leigh-Phippard, mental health service user and carer representative, teacher and scholar, for her overview of this edition and helpful comments made from a patient and public involvement perspective. Finally, we are grateful to Drs Nina Dunne and Chris Cocking for their respective contributions to Chapter 6, on communication and interpersonal skills needed for nurses working with young children, and adolescents and teenagers.

They would also like to thank the following for permission to reproduce copyright material:

Arnold, E and Boggs, KU, *Interpersonal Relationships: Professional communication skills for nurses.* Adapted Table 4.1 (pp73–74), 'Comparison of social and professional relationships.' Copyright © 2006, Elsevier, London. Reproduced with kind permission of the publishers.

DeVito, JA, *The Interpersonal Communication Book.* Copyright © 2007, Pearson Education Inc., Upper Saddle River, NJ. Adapted chart as Figure 4.1 (p78). Reproduced with kind permission of the publishers.

Hargie, O and Dickson, D, *Skilled Interpersonal Communication: Research, theory and practice.* Copyright © 2004, Routledge, London and New York. Adapted types of self box as Table 4.2 (p79). Reproduced with kind permission of the publishers.

Narayansamy, A, The ACCESS model: a transcultural nursing practice framework (p151). *British Journal of Nursing,* 11(9): 643–650. Copyright © 2002. Material reproduced with kind permission of the *British Journal of Nursing.*

Rose, D and Pevalin, DJ, 'Social class based on occupation' (p153), 'Classification by socio-economic group' (p154), 'Operative categories of the National Statistics: Socio-economic Classification (NS-SEC)' (pp154–155), all adapted from *The National Statistics Socio-economic Classification: Origins, development and use.* Institute for Social and Economic Research, University of Essex. Basingstoke: Palgrave Macmillan. Reproduced with kind permission of the publishers.

Every effort has been made to trace all copyright holders within the book, but if any have been inadvertently overlooked, the publisher will be pleased to make the necessary arrangements at the first opportunity.

Introduction

Who is this book for?

This book is primarily intended for first-year degree students of nursing who will inevitably engage with increasingly complex workplace social encounters throughout their course. These encounters will test, hone and, hopefully, gradually improve their *communication and interpersonal skills* (from this point on, the acronym CIPS will be used for convenience). The focus is not to develop knowledge related to any one specific field (Adult, Child, Mental Health or Learning Disabilities), but to support development for progress into any field and beyond. The Nursing and Midwifery Council's *Standards for Pre-registration Nursing Education* (NMC, 2010), as they pertain to CIPS, are a foundation for the book, although its content is not narrowly defined by these standards.

Why CIPS for nursing?

The fact that we have learned since birth how to express ourselves within our family and friendship groups may lead us to take our ability to communicate for granted. Throughout our lives we have been honing our relationship skills, through trial-and-error learning or in response to role modelling by influential others. This may result in us making the assumption that there is no need to think very deeply about how we perform these skills. However, although our practice of interpersonal communication has become second nature, there are times when we have experienced interactions that have not gone smoothly. Perhaps we were misunderstood or friends reacted in ways other than expected. At times like these, we may think that we could have said or done something differently that might have improved our responses and those of people around us. All of this indicates that, while we have developed communication skills, we can always learn and improve when it comes to human relationships. This is mainly because there are so many factors influencing how we might behave in various human encounters, especially encounters in our working lives.

Although similar in some respects to everyday social encounters, the interpersonal context of healthcare work places more of a demand on us to take a developing professional attitude to CIPS. The need for sensitive and professionally executed interpersonal skills is crucial in the overlapping and frequently shifting contexts of healthcare policy, clinical and care environments, and hierarchies of responsibility, not least in the face of human suffering. This backdrop hopefully indicates that the practice of CIPS for developing healthcare professionals places greater and more complex interpersonal challenges on us than when we communicate or interact with family or friends. This highlights the importance of a professional lifetime learning of increasingly effective communication in healthcare settings, and the related challenge of learning to become more aware of ourselves and others.

Unfortunately, there is ample literature to suggest that healthcare staff do not communicate as well as they might in their work settings, thus failing to accord CIPS the degree of seriousness and respect the area deserves. This book, therefore, fulfils an important function, helping you to explore the many factors that impact on communication and relating well to patients, clients, relatives and other healthcare staff. Our overall aim in writing the book is to help you improve your own CIPS.

A word on terminology: the terms 'patient', 'client', 'service user', 'user of . . .' and 'survivor' will be employed variously, to refer to and describe people engaged in nursing and related health-care, as contextually appropriate throughout the book. These are not innocent and equivalent words, as they each carry different assumptions about the appropriate place of people seeking and receiving help and interventions within healthcare cultures (Speed, 2011). This complexity of terminology has related implications for nurses around the style and function of their inter-personal relationships with the public they serve. For example, the word 'patient' can both denote (describe) and connote (imply) people who are the passive recipients of largely biomed-ically driven treatment and care. The interpersonal context shifts with the terms 'service user' or 'user' (of services) and 'client'. These terms can signify persons who are active participants and consumers in their treatment and care, thus suggesting more of a collaborative and equal relationship between them and nurses within mainstream services.

In contrast, the term 'survivor' is often used by people, mostly in a mental health context, who actively resist aspects of roles of both the passive patient and the active consumer of healthcare. In a sustained critique of what they regard as both biomedical reductionism carried out in the name of 'treatment' and 'care', and abuses perpetrated by institutional psychiatry, 'survivors' frequently locate themselves in opposition to aspects of mainstream health services (see, for example, Grant and Leigh-Phippard, 2014).

The main interpersonal implication emerging from this position is the need for mental health nurses, and others, to recognise and work with such people in non-defensive ways. This places a demand on nurses to engage helpfully in relationships where 'recovery' is framed in personally developmental and existential, rather than medicalised, terms. In those contexts, nurses need to respect the desires of people to develop their lives and identities in ways that are independent, and rejecting, of what they perceive to be control, compliance and abuse agendas in mainstream institutional psychiatric practice (Rapley et al., 2011; Grant and Leigh-Phippard, 2014).

Book structure

Chapter 1 introduces the international and national policy and educational context for the nursing practice of CIPS, including the Nursing and Midwifery Council (NMC) *Standards for Pre-registration Nursing Education* (2010). Against this backdrop, the key concepts of the book are unpacked and defined, and their relevance for the student nurse from the first day of training is stressed. Some theoretical communication frameworks are explained, as is the relationship between CIPS and the domains of caring, moral practice, suffering, healthy relating and empathy in nursing.

Chapter 2 covers some of the key issues in the evidence base underpinning the practice of CIPS in nursing. It begins by summarising the general benefits of the sensitive practice of CIPS emerging from research on CIPS directly, and from relevant principles emerging from psychotherapy research. The discussion then turns to the historical development of CIPS research in nursing in the context of evidence-based healthcare. Evidence-based healthcare is first discussed in conventional terms, where biomedical, quantitative-experimental research is privileged, and then with regard to more contemporary claims to what constitutes 'evidence' from the 'lived experience' paradigm. It is stressed that the practice of CIPS is inextricably context-bound, in that it is always embedded in time, place, the specific form of the relationship of the communicators and the organisational frameworks within which communication takes place. Given this, it will be argued that many healthcare environments currently demand briefer forms of CIPS rather than extended forms drawn from counselling and psychotherapy models. Deriving in large part from Rogerian therapy, these models are subjected to an extended critique throughout the chapter. The discussion also focuses on the importance of understanding the development and exercise of schemas and, in related terms, stereotyping and prejudice. The relevance of the concepts of first- and second-level communication is stressed, and there is a discussion of some of the difficulties in teaching empathy to nurses. Finally, organisational threats to the practice of CIPS in nursing are discussed.

Chapter 3 emphasises the importance of the *safe* and *effective* practice of CIPS underpinned by social thinking processes. The chapter explores the many roles you will have in relation to CIPS, and the core general skills that are needed in its practice. The phases of the nurse–patient relationship are discussed in relation to two models. The nature of the helping relationship in nursing is examined and it is argued that this relationship can have a therapeutic effect. Finally, the patient's role in decision making in the nurse–patient relationship is analysed in relation to recent health policy.

Chapter 4 discusses the factors that act as barriers and impede effective communication and interpersonal relationships. It begins by investigating the shift you are required to make in your professional work when you move from social to safe professional relationships. It does so by examining the different degrees of intimacy between friend and carer, and the rules of social engagement. The discussion then turns to the effect that emotions can have on communication and interpersonal relationships. Other barriers to communication are then explored, including how people construct meaning and interpret communication as a function of this construction. The effect of motivation on communicating health advice is also examined. The chapter concludes by considering the nature of conflict, what causes it and how it can be diffused in healthcare situations.

Chapter 5 helps you to examine what will be involved in your continuing needs as a lifelong learner. Some of the issues around the integration of theory and practice are explored, in relation to ways in which learning should be realistic and relevant to your practice and learning needs. Learning CIPS through experience, or learning by doing, will be emphasised. A framework for levels of academic qualifications is presented with a discussion on how this links to practice. The skills deriving from examining this framework will enable you to operate more effectively within complex care environments for decision making, and will facilitate problem solving, critical thinking and reflective capacities. Links will be made with the assessment of practice requirements to enable you to have a clearer idea of how to gain proficiency in skills. The sections on reflective writing, learning styles and the characteristics of a skilled performance will help you complete your practice learning assessments in relation to the use of CIPS in your practice learning experiences. Some guidelines are provided for improving communication in relation to some of the different contexts in which you can act as an educator with colleagues and patients. The final section of the chapter looks to your future as a lifelong learner of CIPS.

Chapter 6 examines the environmental context of CIPS. It begins with a discussion on the importance of CIPS within multidisciplinary team practice and interprofessional working, across different care settings and within safe environments. The chapter then turns to the ways in which physical and social-environmental factors shape communication, in relation to working with different populations. In this context, it will be argued that power is utilised to the advantage of some groups and the disadvantage of others. Next, the interrelated concepts of prejudice and schema development (first introduced in Chapter 2) are further explored. These concepts are extremely important in understanding how CIPS can break down in specific healthcare environmental contexts. The discussion then explores the impact of shifting friendship, family and cultural networks on communication and interpersonal behaviour and skill development. The demands on CIPS arising from British multicultural society are contrasted with institutional racism and its impact on communication in healthcare environments. The chapter ends with a critique of the tendency emerging from humanistic psychology to view CIPS as solely located within the individual. In the light of the preceding argument, it is argued that this 'fallacy of individualism' conveys a naive and overly optimistic picture of human interaction.

Chapter 7 begins with a focus on the interpersonal and ethical contexts of nursing people from different backgrounds and cultures. It begins with a discussion of immigration and migration to help you understand how diverse ethnic populations in many of our neighbourhoods in the UK have developed, and the motivators for migration. The chapter then explores CIPS in the context of cultural diversity by examining concepts such as cultural preservation, negotiation and repatterning, or restructuring. Some of the issues of nursing in a multicultural Britain and the need for cultural awareness and cultural competence are examined, and two theories of transcultural care are compared. The discussion then turns to diversity and socio-economic position, in relation to a society that is made up of different groups to which power, influence and opportunities are not always equally granted. The chapter concludes with a section that considers the ethical and moral consequences of communication and personal interactions.

Chapter 8 brings the book to a close. With an eye to your future, it will help you situate the practice of CIPS in nursing 'beyond technique' within a set of interlinked professional developmental, cultural, social-organisational, political and moral concerns. Specifically, you will be invited to consider the context of CIPS in critically reflective professional development, where 'technical rationality' is contrasted with 'professional artistry'. It will be argued that this consideration has implications for social relationships in healthcare practice in that exclusively technical rational approaches to CIPS in nursing practice may arguably undermine and trivialise their worth.

The sustained practice of critical reflexivity will be promoted in contrast, as a means of helping you maintain fidelity with high-quality CIPS practice and awareness in your future career, in the context of professional artistry.

There is a glossary of key terms at the end of the book. Terms included will appear in **bold** type the first time they are mentioned.

NMC *Standards for Pre-registration Nursing Education* and Essential Skills Clusters

The NMC has standards of competence that have to be met by applicants to different parts of the nursing and midwifery register. These standards are what the NMC deems are necessary for the delivery of safe, effective nursing and midwifery practice.

As well as specific competencies, the NMC identifies specific skills that nursing students must have at various points of their training programme. These Essential Skills Clusters (ESCs) are essential abilities that students need to attain in order to practise to their full potential. This book identifies some of the competencies and skills, within the realm of reflective practice, that student nurses need in order to be entered on to the NMC register. These competencies and ESCs are presented at the start of each chapter so that it is clear which of them the chapter addresses. All of the competencies and ESCs in this book relate to the *generic standards* that all nursing students must achieve. This book includes the latest standards, taken from the *Standards for Pre-registration Nursing Education* (NMC, 2010).

The generic standard for competence, which applies throughout the book, states that:

> *All nurses must use excellent communication and interpersonal skills. Their communications must always be safe, effective, compassionate and respectful. Nurses must communicate effectively using a wide range of strategies and interventions, including the effective use of communication technologies. Where people have a disability, nurses must be able to work with service users and others to obtain the information needed to make reasonable adjustments that promote optimum health and enable equal access to services.*
> (NMC, 2010, p24)

Activities

At various stages within each chapter there are points at which you can break to undertake activities. Undertaking and understanding the activities are important elements of your understanding of the content of each chapter. You are encouraged, where appropriate, to reflect on your practice and consider how the things you have learned from working with patients might inform your understanding of reflection and reflective practice. Other activities will require you to take time away from the book to find out new information that will add to your understanding of the topic under discussion. Some activities challenge you to apply your learning to a question or scenario to help you reflect on issues and practice in more depth. A few activities require you to make observations during your day-to-day life or in the clinical setting. All these activities are designed to increase your understanding of the topics under discussion and how they reflect on nursing practice.

Remember, academic study will always require independent work; attending lectures will never be enough to be successful on your programme, and these activities will help to deepen your knowledge and understanding of the issues under scrutiny and give you practice at working on your own.

Chapter 1
Understanding communication and interpersonal skills

NMC Standards for Pre-registration Nursing Education

This chapter will address the following competencies:

Domain 2: Communication and interpersonal skills

3. All nurses must use the full range of communication methods, including verbal, non-verbal and written, to acquire, interpret and record their knowledge and understanding of people's needs. They must be aware of their own values and beliefs and the impact this may have on their communication with others. They must take account of the many different ways in which people communicate and how these may be influenced by ill health, disability and other factors, and be able to recognise and respond effectively when a person finds it hard to communicate.

6. All nurses must take every opportunity to encourage health-promoting behaviour through education, role modelling and effective communication.

NMC Essential Skills Clusters

This chapter will address the following ESCs:

Cluster: Care, compassion and communication

1. As partners in the care process, people can trust a newly registered graduate nurse to provide collaborative care based on the highest standards, knowledge and competence.

By the first progression point:

1. Articulates the underpinning values of *The Code: Standards of conduct, performance and ethics for nurses and midwives (The Code)* (NMC, 2008).
2. Works within limitations of the role and recognises own level of competence.

By the second progression point:

6. Forms appropriate and constructive professional relationships with families and other carers.

> ## Chapter aims
>
> By the end of this chapter, you should be able to:
>
> - understand the importance of student nurses making their own assessment of their CIPS, at the start of their pre-registration training programme;
> - appreciate the importance of CIPS in relation to national and international nursing policy and educational literature;
> - describe communication frameworks governing CIPS;
> - understand the relationship between CIPS and caring, moral practice, suffering, and healthy relating in nursing;
> - have an adequate platform from which to develop your knowledge, and related skills, about empathy in CIPS, and its function in humanising nursing care.

Introduction

From very early times, when human beings began to evolve and cohabit in an environment that was both hostile and primitive, a crucial early skill that emerged and took hold, essential to the survival and development of our species, was the **communication** of ideas. This enabled people to share understandings, protect one another and develop new ways of solving the problems they encountered in their everyday lives in order to survive. We can also hazard a guess that, after a while, they were communicating facts about where to find the best berries or tracks of the nearest herd of woolly mammoths. Gradually, they began to be able to express humour, rage, excitement, fear, desire and jealousy. With the development of emotional and aesthetic sophistication, we can imagine times when they sighed in mutual appreciation over a beautiful sunset or wondered about shooting stars. Communication abilities linked with social collaboration enabled them to identity the best and worst places to hunt and the value of one animal fur garment over another.

So that a transfer of information between each other could be more easily understood by early humans, different forms of communication emerged, including the development of language. Methods of communication for language in the written and spoken form have continued to evolve over the millennia to the extent that, in our present world, we are using highly technological methods such as the internet and other electronic formats.

In relation to the kinship groups and social networks evidenced by anthropological evidence, these evolved refinements would have developed from, and been based around, the connectedness of the individuals and their relationships. These basic premises have not changed for us in our current day-to-day activities. The means of communication may have advanced and become more varied and technical, but the basic human need to communicate and share ideas with those we know, work with or care for has not changed.

In this chapter we will begin by emphasising how important it is that you begin to assess your own CIPS, given that you will be expected to use and develop these skills from the start of your nurse preparation programme. We will provide some practical case and clinical scenarios based on what a first-year student may expect to encounter in exercising these skills. We will then explore international and national policy and educational literature pertaining to CIPS, before attempting to unpack and define associated concepts, including the crucial importance of empathy. The chapter will conclude with a discussion on the organisational basis for the practice of CIPS.

The importance of CIPS for the first-year student nurse

In Annexe 2 of the *Standards for Pre-registration Nursing Education*, the NMC (2010, p98) describes the first progression point criteria. These are the *Criteria that must be met as a minimum requirement by progression point one in any practice setting where people are receiving care, or through simulation*. In relation to the competency domain of *communication and **interpersonal skills***, these criteria consist of:

- safety and safeguarding people of all ages, their carers and their families;
- professional values and expected attitudes and behaviours towards people, their carers and their families.

So, right from the start of your nurse education, you will be expected to use CIPS to demonstrate that you are able in your practice to ensure the safety of the patients you work with, and their carers and families. You will be expected to demonstrate this within an appropriate set of nursing values, and related attitudes and behaviours.

How does this translate into CIPS knowledge and practice? This question will be explored throughout this book. For the moment, let us consider a single scenario with two different outcomes, demonstrating poor and good practice respectively, in relation to the communication and competency domain for the first progression point criteria. We ask you to imagine that you are the student nurse in this scenario.

Scenario: A distressed patient

Jenny is on the first day of her first practice experience in the first year of her nursing education. The only nurse on this particular part of the ward, she notices a small group of relatives gathered around an elderly female patient. The relatives are talking in raised voices and the patient appears distressed by this. Jenny had been asked by the staff nurse on duty to carry out a specific task, involving collecting equipment in another area of the ward. Because she wants to make a good impression on her first day, she wants to carry out this task as quickly as possible so decides to do nothing about the scenario she has just witnessed.

Scenario: Responding to a patient's distress

Susan is on the first day of her first practice experience in the first year of her nursing education. The only nurse on this particular part of the ward, she notices a small group of relatives gathered around an elderly female patient. The relatives are talking in raised voices and the patient appears distressed by this. Susan had been asked by the staff nurse on duty to carry out a specific task, involving collecting equipment in another area of the ward. Although she wants to make a good impression with her new colleagues, she is equally aware of the need to prioritise the care and safety needs of the patient. Despite feeling anxious about her decision and its possible consequences, she interrupts the task she was involved in to report what she has witnessed to the nurse in charge. The nurse in charge responds quickly and tactfully intervenes with the relatives and patient to try to find out what the problem is, in order to facilitate its resolution as quickly as possible.

Consider the differences between the two outcomes of the scenario in relation to the first progression point criteria and related communication competency domains described above. In the first outcome, Jenny prioritised routine tasks over the need to safeguard the people in her care and their relatives. By choosing this line of action, she failed in her duty to communicate this event properly to the senior nurse on the ward. Finally, by placing her own need to be well thought of over the needs of her patient and relatives, she demonstrated unprofessional values, attitudes and behaviour. In the second outcome, in contrast, Susan properly interrupted the task that was delegated to her in order to communicate what she had witnessed promptly, without going beyond her range of expertise, knowledge and status.

Activity 1.1   *Evidence-based practice and research*

Log on to the NMC website and enter the title 'Standards for Pre-registration Nursing Education'. Read through the standards and competencies for 'Communication and interpersonal skills' and the ESCs for 'Care, compassion and communication'. Clarify the level of CIPS needed for you in your training, in relation to progression points.

Hint: This activity will develop your knowledge and awareness of CIPS in relation to your nursing training, and beyond.

International and national policy on CIPS

Reflected in the NMC *Standards for Pre-registration Nursing Education* (2010), the World Health Organization (2000b), European Union (2004), Department of Health (DH) (2004) and the National Health Service (NHS) Modernisation Agency (2003) have all emphasised the importance of patient-focused communication between health professionals and patients. This is seen as vital to achieving patient satisfaction, inclusive decision making in caregiving and an efficient health service.

Recent emphasis on dignity and respect from the DH, and professional bodies such as the Royal College of Nursing and NMC, has highlighted the issues for sections of the public that have not received quality care from health professionals. The Dignity in Care Campaign aims to end tolerance of indignity in health and social care services through raising awareness and inspiring people to take action (see useful websites at the end of this chapter). Older people and people with mental health and/or learning disabilities have been highlighted as care groups that require special attention in healthcare services for personalised care. The role of person-centred care and CIPS is integral to the accommodation of these care groups.

In a similar vein, the *Essence of Care* series has been designed by the DH to support the measures to improve quality, and will contribute to the introduction of clinical governance at local levels. The benchmarking process outlined in the *Essence of Care* (NHS Modernisation Agency, 2003) helps practitioners to take a structured approach to sharing and comparing practice, enabling them to identify the best and to develop action plans to remedy poor practice. *Essence of Care* benchmarks for communication have been produced for clinical governance, promoting health and the care environment (see useful websites at the end of this chapter).

Activity 1.2 — *Reflection*

Recall a care setting that you have visited recently and think about the levels of dignity and respect given to the patients or clients in that setting. Would you consider that there needs to be improvement? If yes, identify what you consider wrong with existing levels of dignity and respect given to patients, how you think things should change and the possible barriers to achieving this change.

Hint: This activity will develop your ability to evaluate the practice of CIPS in different healthcare environments, and will prepare you for some of the challenges to the practice of effective and skilled CIPS in nursing that you will read about throughout this book.

Key issues from the nursing literature and CIPS

Nursing literature also promotes the above concepts as indicative of best practice (for example, McCabe and Timmins, 2006, 2013; NMC, 2010). Charlton et al. (2008) found that, by using an approach that prioritised the needs of the patient in the interaction between nurses and patients or clients, care outcomes were improved in:

- patient satisfaction;
- adherence to treatment options;
- patient health.

However, there is some evidence to suggest that, while qualified nurses often rate their own communication skills as high, patients report less satisfaction and maintain that communication could be improved. In addition, there is evidence that some nurses stereotype patient groups. In other words, they give them a blanket label as a group and then act towards each individual in the group as if that label were true (Timmins, 2007).

There are criticisms of teaching CIPS in nursing education that point to a lack of systematic evaluation of such teaching and a difficulty in resolving the difference between the school way and the ward way internationally (Chant et al., 2002; Shields et al., 2012; Stanley et al., 2014). There is thus a need to consider learning these skills in the clinical environment with greater involvement of clinical staff. The aim of this book is therefore to contribute to the learning of CIPS, to give students an opportunity to think about their own CIPS and to seek opportunities to practise achieving their CIPS learning outcomes in the practice environment.

Effective communication is also essential to both practice and improving interpersonal relationships in the workplace between professional groups and peers (Grover, 2005). It is acknowledged that successful communication is shaped by basic techniques, such as open-ended questions, listening, **empathy** and assertiveness. However, successful interpersonal relationships are also affected by a number of factors. These include beliefs professionals have about the status and significance of their profession, gender, generation, environmental context and collegiality, and beliefs about cooperation, self-disclosure and reciprocity. These can impede or enhance the outcome of quality communication, depending on how CIPS is understood and defined.

Defining and understanding CIPS

There are many texts written for nurses that seek to explain CIPS. Definitions in the therapeutic communication skills literature generally vary from the apparently highly technical and impersonal to the more human. Consider the following examples that span several decades and make a decision about the one or ones that appeal to you most, and the reasons for its/their appeal.

Communication is about the reciprocal process in which messages are sent and received between two or more people.
(Balzer-Riley, 2004)

Interpersonal communication involves a series of messages or information which people send out to, and receive from, each other through the use of the senses, such as seeing, touching and hearing one another.
(Petrie, 1997)

Communication is a universal function of humankind, independent of any place, time or context.
(Ruesch, 1961)

What kinds of factors influenced your choice? Is communication between people, or interpersonal communication, simply and only a functional part of life, undertaken to get things done? Or is communication, in addition to its practical purposes, more about enriching the quality of our lives as individuals and in groups?

I don't need to work at developing communication and interpersonal skills. They come naturally.

This is a commonly expressed view among some students new to nursing. How true is it? Read the following paragraphs on communication frameworks and then ask yourself this question again.

Communication frameworks

Communication is considered a basic tool in healthcare relationships. However, the quality of the communication has a strong relationship to its effectiveness. Two useful theoretical models which may help us to achieve a good understanding of how communication takes place are the linear and the circular, or transactional, models. The linear model involves communication from a sender to a receiver via a message (Table 1.1). The message is relayed by one or more of the five senses (sight, touch, hearing, taste or smell).

Sender →	Message →	Receiver
Idea is encoded and expressed Sender has the responsibility for accuracy of the content and emotional tone	Verbal and/or non-verbal thoughts and/or feelings	Idea is decoded, translated into words or symbols and made sense of

Table 1.1: Linear framework of communication

A more modern addition to this rather simplistic model is to consider communication as a circular rather than linear process, and a process that takes account of a larger social system and context. The model was originally developed by Bateson (1979), and is still relevant today as it takes account of the effects of the context within which an interaction takes place. Communication is viewed as being continuous, involving mutual giving and receiving. It is an expansion of the linear model and uses a systems approach to understanding communication. In systems models, each part has an effect on another part in the system. The sender and receiver each has a set of characteristics that influence the communication. There are shared characteristics for both, which are: culture, knowledge, communication abilities and style, values, internal frame of reference and role. The sender has a set of factors that relate to his or her needs and goals, and the sender's communication style and abilities influence the communication. The receiver also has goals and needs, but added to this are the receiver's previous experiences and any support systems that he or she may have or will have (Figure 1.1).

This model emphasises the complexity of communication and the many factors that have to be taken into account. It also indicates that the ability of the communicator has a significant effect and the internal value systems of the individuals involved in communicating with each other play a part. There is also a strong hint in this model that it is not just communicating that enables messages to be transmitted. The interpersonal nature of one person's response to another person counts. The situational context in which the interaction takes place also has an effect.

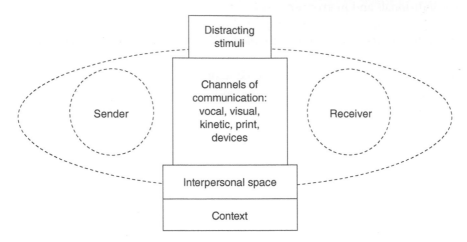

Figure 1.1: Circular transactional framework of communication

Fundamental concepts in communication and interpersonal skills

The meaning of the concept of 'communication' can be simply stated as the exchange of information between people by means of speaking, writing or using a common system of signs or behaviour. The 'interpersonal' concept refers to the connection between two or more people or groups and their involvement with one another, especially with regard to the way they behave towards and feel about one another.

Theory summary: What is a concept?

In general, it is accepted that a concept is a broad theoretical idea that someone has thought up, or named, to help us picture how an intangible idea can be understood and to enable us to express this idea through language. To take this discussion one step further, concepts are also deemed to be abstract, that is, not concrete, but expressing a quality, emotion or thought, and thus something you cannot necessarily see or touch. A concept can also be deemed a principle that guides somebody's actions, especially one that has a value or importance attached to the ideas, to be followed as a guide for human behaviours and responses. Exploring concepts is a means of describing and analysing incidents, and a technique used extensively in this book to capture the meaning of how, for example, people's behaviour is perceived and understood in relation to events.

It would be helpful to consider the difference between the two concepts of 'communication' and 'interpersonal skills' and why we have brought them together in this book. Exchanging information through the communication of ideas, fact and emotions is a complex phenomenon, and cannot take place in nursing without the recognition of the many context-specific factors that influence the communication. Communication, as you will discover in subsequent chapters, requires many different methods and processes to become effective. Even when we are not speaking or writing, and invoking silence instead, we are still communicating a message with a meaning that will need to be interpreted. Consequently, all forms of communication need interpreting, and the factors influencing communication need to be accounted for.

The relationship between 'communication' and 'interpersonal skills'

Well-practised communication techniques alone are ineffectual if the central notion of the interpersonal connection goes unacknowledged. In the nursing context, the primary factor is the relationship between nurse and patient or service user, co-worker, relatives or carers. We are unlikely to communicate without some form of relationship, whether through an information leaflet or poster where there is an intention to relate to persons who may or may not be known, or by physically being close to a person in a bed or chair who is in need of support to prevent suffering, or through a lifesaving intervention or information to prevent further deterioration of a health-related problem.

In this light, Charlton et al. (2008) differentiated between two different communication styles in the literature they reviewed. These were biomedical and biopsychosocial. The biomedical style concentrated on giving specific information on details concerning the patient's condition and was information-focused. The biopsychosocial style was identified as patient-centred communication and this style had a more demonstrable impact on patient outcomes.

Jones (2007) maintains that there is little research in nursing literature that discusses interpersonal skills, particularly in nursing education, whereas there is a rich supply of communication skills research and literature. This is despite research and policy that have promoted patient-centred communication as effective. There is also a critique that nursing education is often removed from the realities that students experience during their practice learning experiences (Shields et al., 2012), which points to the lack of literature on CIPS in nursing situations in the clinical environment.

Essential communication skills are deemed to be listening and attending, empathy, information giving and support in the context of a **helping relationship**. The focus needs to be person-centred rather than nurse- or task-focused, and the relationship is a key element. Time spent developing this key relationship is an investment and yet often a precious commodity. Busy wards with high-dependency patients are the norm in many acute care settings, but time spent in nurses attempting to understand patients' individual needs is indispensable (McCabe and Timmins, 2006, 2013).

Specific areas of nursing specialty require tailored approaches to CIPS, for example in palliative care, in care of the dying, or with children, persons with mental health problems, physical disabilities or learning difficulties. Equally, different settings, such as accident and emergency or intensive care, long-stay wards, and clinics and community settings, will all require different or particular approaches to CIPS. It is the responsibility of the nurse to identify where these specific needs may be. There is literature and research available in all these areas of practice. A good habit to develop is familiarity with literature searching so that you can find the resources you need to help you with specific settings or care groups. Some of these areas will be covered later in this book, illustrated by case studies. You may be dealing with individuals or groups, for short or long periods of time and in intense emotional situations or circumstances where emotional distance is required. The variety and range of situations are almost infinite.

This discussion so far implies that there are varying forms of interpersonal proximity and degrees of intensity, purpose and significance that make up the interpersonal aspects of communication in nursing. We are using communication methods from the moment we are born, beginning with the intimacy of the parent–infant interaction, through to the more diffuse connections we have with social networks or in public places such as on the bus each morning travelling to work. Developing our CIPS effectively in different circumstances and with different people has helped us to hone our skills. There is a difference between social and professional situations, as clearly there is more at stake in the latter if we are ineffective with these skills, and it is in the latter that we have to underpin the application of CIPS with caring.

Caring and nursing

Caring is nursing, and nursing is caring.
(Leininger, 1984, p83)

The concept of caring in nursing was a subject of intense interest in the latter decades of the twentieth century (Clarke and Wheeler, 1992; Kyle, 1995). From a perspective that takes into account cultural similarities and differences across individuals and populations, Leininger (1981, 1984) argued that caring in nursing is about the provision of comfort, concern and support, the development of trust and the alleviation of stress. Clearly, whether practised across or within cultures, caring can only be demonstrated when people interact with each other – hence its connection to CIPS.

Interest in conceptualising and defining the concept of caring has developed since the late 1980s. Morse et al. (1991) undertook a detailed analysis of the concept and identified five major areas. These authors saw caring as:

- a human trait;
- a moral imperative;
- an affect;
- an interpersonal interaction;
- a therapeutic intervention.

Radsma (1994), like Leininger (1984) and Brykczynska (1997), considers caring to be an integral component of nursing, although Radsma claims that nurses have a dilemma in explaining and justifying the significance, meaning and function of nursing care because they believe it to be so integral to everything that they do. The studies of Benner and Wrubel (1988), Clarke and Wheeler (1992), Lea et al. (1998) and Kitson (2003) are all examples of empirical research identifying the components of caring actions in nursing, and have helped to articulate what the elements of caring are, in order to bring them into the real world and away from abstract conceptualisation.

Benner et al. (1996) described caring practice in several domains:

- the helping role;
- teaching/coaching functions;
- diagnostic and patient-monitoring functions;
- effective management of rapidly changing situations;
- administering and monitoring therapeutic interventions and regimens.

The above conceptualisation of caring is very different from that described in Watson's (1988) transpersonal theory. This theory is organised around concepts such as transpersonalism, phenomenology, the self and the caring occasion, with ten curative factors that guide nursing care. Watson's theory is intended to encompass the whole of nursing; however, it places most emphasis on the experiential, interpersonal processes between the caregiver and recipient. It focuses on caring as a **therapeutic relationship** and attempts to reduce the components of caring to describable parts, so that these parts can be understood and learned. Watson believes that nursing is *a human-to-human relationship in which the person of nurse affects and is affected by the person of the other* (1988, p58). This might usefully be regarded as *relational caring* (Hartrick, 1997). Hartrick suggests that more emphasis should be placed on relationship development than on skills development.

Caring in practice

Caring in practice (Spichiger et al., 2005) explores the notion of commitment, and the difference between *technical* care that is embedded in practice and *relational* care that attempts to attune itself to actions engaged with others using experience, perceptiveness and an understanding of the responses of others. These ideas spring from developments and debates in nursing theory about the relationship and embeddedness of caring in nursing. So much so that a science of caring is now being accepted as a main stream in nursing education, although less so in the UK.

There have been two main centres for the development of caring science. From the USA has emerged the work of Jean Watson in the 1970s–1990s (Watson, 1997): Watson developed pre-existing nursing theory to place caring at the centre of all nursing activities, decisions and practices. More recently, Watson has proposed that the most important resource in the caring relationship between patient and nurse is healthcare professionals, as it is they who provide the resource to carry out the phenomena of caring. From the Scandinavian countries, the work of Katie Erikson (2002) has been pivotal in defining caring science with a more spiritual and ethical approach to caring underpinned by humanistic thinking, concerned with the interests and welfare of humans, rather than the transpersonal approach and process approach taken by Watson.

While caring is considered to be a core value in nursing, there are only a handful of education curricula in the UK that have internalised caring into programme structures, although concepts may have been taught in seminars and lectures (Brown, 2011). One reason for this is that the notion of caring has been assumed and implicit; that is, until the exposure of exceedingly poor practice in the Winterbourne View care home (DH, 2012) and NHS Mid Staffordshire Hospital (DH, 2012, 2013; Francis, 2013), which highlighted that these aspects of nursing care are not universally evident in nursing practice. This raises the questions of why this form of care has not been made explicit and why it has been assumed to be implicit.

Another reason why caring has not been made more explicit is that is an elusive concept to research and requires qualitative methodologies that have been considered unorthodox and unreliable, such as phenomenology, when compared with research methods that can be tested out against a hypothesis and described in quantifiable terms. There are few who would not agree that it is impossible to capture caring activity that takes place in an environment determined by context, such as a ward or someone's home, in a laboratory and measure it. There have been attempts to do this and Lea et al. (1998) designed a questionnaire (a caring dimensions inventory) and, while this was tested in a limited number of clinical environments, it did not become adopted extensively. The questionnaire was aimed at measuring perceptions of caring and found that these were framed as technical attributes of care and their characteristics developed as the students progressed through their programmes. Yet Murphy et al. (2009) found, when studying student nurses during the three-year period of their course, that they became inured to caring behaviours, and third-year students scored lower than first-year students on the questionnaire.

In a study of caring and culture in the clinical areas, Ousey and Johnson (2007) found that students assumed that fundamental and emotional care was the role of healthcare workers. The changing boundaries of medical and nursing professional care and responsibilities for care added to this situation. Maben et al. (2007b) suggested that student nurses revealed that, prior to qualifying, they had high ideals about how they would like to care for patients. Students were followed up 4–6 and 11–15 months later once they were qualified. They spoke of those nurses they did not want to emulate, who considered nursing 'just a job' and were not good caring role models. They gave examples of ways they tried to make a difference. Over 70 per cent of these nurses then described how this work was undermined, undervalued and not valued in comparison to task-oriented aspects of the work. Maben uncovered a set of covert rules which, together with overwhelming organisational constraints, relentlessly hampered their nursing ideals. These unwritten rules included hurried physical care, 'don't get involved with patients', 'fit in and don't try to change practice'. The studies in the examples given above indicate that potentially caring behaviours become less important over time in a student nurse's life and are affected by their experiences in practice. There is room to examine again what the elements are in a caring relationship so that they are sustained in caring situations beyond the students' course years and continue into practice over the lifetime of the nurse career and working life.

There are examples of research where it has been attempted to capture what could be described as the elements of elusive and intangible caring concepts, and the work of Bach (2004) is one of the few examples. Bach (2004) researched the relationship between psychology and caring. She found that there were distinct characteristics that patients found nurses provided, in what nurses described as 'psychological care'. These characteristics were deemed to be similar to some of the therapeutic activities of formal psychological care provided by trained therapists. Moreover, Bach found that the interpersonal relationship between the nurse and patient was crucial to carrying out psychological care. To explain what these characteristics are, and how they might be recognised as part of the psychological caring process in nursing, a model was designed. The characteristics identified in the research are part of the hidden or unseen aspects of psychological care as opposed to physical or observable characteristics. The aim was to illustrate the characteristic activities of psychological care in a representational model using a prism that refracts, is usually transparent and is a parallelogram (representing both pairs of opposite sides as parallel in the nurse–patient relationship; Figure 1.2).

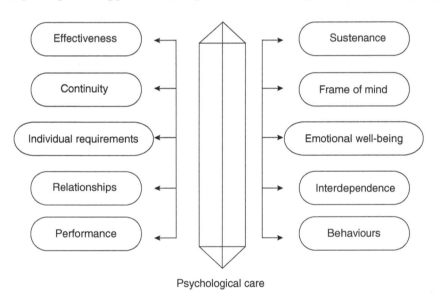

Figure 1.2: Psychological care

The notion that caring is invisible, but 'felt' or experienced by both parties in the relationship, is not new. Watson's (1988) transpersonal theory also features this phenomenon; however, Bach (2004) identified the characteristics that nurses described in the psychological caring relationship. These characteristics were corroborated by patients from a variety of nursing settings, which helped to define the elements of nurse–patient interactions. The process of describing the characteristics helps to understand how the abstract, or hidden, elements can become tangible or seen and consequently are more easily integrated into practice by those learning to care for patients in this manner or to enhance care given by qualified practitioners. To help understand the features underpinning each characteristic, the following gives a brief overview.

- *Interdependence* is the interaction between physical, psychological, social and economic situations and the impact of cultural, generational and environmental influences on patients' lives.

- *Dynamic relationships between patient and nurse* are processes of engagement, requiring negotiating skills and the ability to engage on different levels.

- *Performance of non-visible care* involves alleviating psychological distress, being humane, giving peace of mind and giving patients/clients a sense of control over their bodies as well as their minds. It involves building rapport, being observant and estimating how patients/clients perceive and respond to their worlds. It is being respectful, watchful, empowering and recognising vulnerability and unreality, and being sensitive towards patients' distress, giving encouragement, enabling problem solving, engendering confidence, providing distraction from distress and proffering solutions that are based on psychological knowledge.

- *Continuity* means continually processing, assessing and collecting information on which to base an understanding of the patients' situations. Time spent with patients to achieve this could be momentary or ongoing and vary according to staffing levels. Initial assessments are important, however, and information is continuously amended to provide continuing care.

- *Frame or state of mind* is a repository view of the mind where cognitive processes such as thoughts, levels of intelligence, information and motivations are arranged and managed by the individual. The effects of this state of mind influence behaviours and the nurse's role is to look after this state of mind.

- *Emotional well-being* involves caring for emotional and mental well-being, observing emotional instability and stability and, most of all, giving emotional support. It is dealing with the emotional consequences of the state of mind and giving time to people to explore their feelings and have some release from their stored-up worries and emotions.

- *Human behaviours and actions* concern the role of human behaviours, actions and reactions. Try to understand the potential, and actual, psychological context and consequences of these behaviours. Observe and note, with the intention of addressing the psychological implications in relation to behavioural responses.

- *Individuality* in the form of individualised care is paramount. Some people need more psychological support than others and some only need psychological care.

- *Effectiveness* is not merely an emphasis on processes such as listening and supporting. Patients felt that this type of care gives confirmation to them that what they were doing, and how they felt and reacted, was acceptable and that they were being taken seriously. It involves helping to find answers, a sense of security and comfort, helping people through transitions, and supporting them on their life journeys – a sense that the nurses believed in them. It is creating a feel-good factor that induces a sense of self-esteem and self-efficacy.

- *Sustenance* involves different forms of support such as to maintain, continue and sustain daily life over a period of time, which in turn enables patients to sustain their psychological strength.

Activity 1.3   *Critical thinking*

Can you remember an encounter with someone you knew and who you were caring for?

- Describe the components of that encounter from both your own and the other person's perspective. Use the model in Figure 1.2 to guide you. Are they similar?
- Compare this with an encounter with someone you did not know. What differences did you find between the two encounters? For example, what information did you take for granted about both the person you knew and the person you did not know? What was the difference between the two sets of information?

Hint: This activity will help you evaluate the differences between encounters based on personal knowledge of the other and impersonal knowledge. It will also help you in using your imagination to think and feel what it must be like from the other person's perspective – a necessary skill in the development of empathy.

Lifelong learning and CIPS

The NMC *Standards for Pre-registration Nursing Education* (2010) stress that nurses should commit themselves to lifelong learning, to extend the scope of their professional practice safely and effectively and to think in a future-directed and nursing field-related way.

According to the NMC, this commitment should be made within the full range of, often highly different, multidisciplinary team workplaces. These workplaces should promote safety and responsiveness to the needs of the patients/clients within them.

What would a commitment to these standards mean for the healthcare organisations, and the nurses working in them, that were sensitive to the need for the development of increasingly effective and sophisticated interpersonal communication for nurses and midwives? Writers such as Benner et al. (cited in Frost et al., 2000), for example, argue that CIPS are on just as much a continuum from 'novice' to 'expert' as are technical nursing skills. Benner and colleagues argue that highly proficient nurses demonstrate the ability for 'emotional attunement' with their clients. In the context of safe, effective and compassionate organisational work settings, this means that:

> *Attuned nurses have a capacity to read a situation in a patient and to grasp its emotional tone: to know when something is 'off' when it looks 'ok' on the surface, or to sense that it's actually 'ok' despite appearances to the contrary.*
> (Frost et al., 2000, p32)

> ### Case study: Attunement
>
> *A community nurse visits one of her patients to dress her leg ulcer. She does this on a regular basis and usually finds her patient cheerful and engaging. On this particular day, however, she notices that her patient, although apparently pleasant and cheerful as usual, seems 'off'. The nurse doesn't receive any obvious signs to tell her that something is wrong with her patient, but has a 'gut feeling' that something is not right. She is used to trusting and acting on such instinct, even though she can't rationally articulate its nature or why she trusts it. She spends more time than usual with her patient and, over a cup of tea, sensitively and gently questions her about what might be wrong. The patient discloses that her husband has recently become unwell with suspected heart problems. This has been worrying her since the nurse's last visit.*

To help improve our CIPS, theorists have explored the manner in which we communicate and relate to one another to provide us with explanations for why and how we carry out what could be considered a fundamental human behaviour. Because there are so many different factors that can affect our ability to communicate, we will be concentrating in the sections that follow on the following crucial aspects: **moral practice**, **suffering** and **healthy relating**.

Moral practice

CIPS need to be worked on over the lifespan of a nursing career, within organisations that truly deserve the title of caring. In the facilitation of this, several nurse scholar-practitioners and scholars from disciplines other than nursing have, over the years, provided a theoretical foundation that is arguably indispensable. The strands of this foundation illustrate a concern for the ongoing, ethically important development of 'moral' practice (Armstrong, 2006; Clay and Povey, 1983; Wurzbach, 1999). Quite simply, moral practice amounts to believing that 'good' and 'right' practice is to be desired over practice that is 'bad' and 'wrong'. Moral practice demands that we develop sensitivity to the suffering of others.

Suffering

Interpersonal sensitivity, used in the service of helping others within a trusting relationship, must be linked to a sensitivity to the suffering of others. From a review of the literature, undertaken to help nurses gain a better conceptual understanding of this area, Rodgers and Cowles (1997) argued that suffering is a complex concept that cannot be readily observed or measured. According to these authors, its individual and subjective nature means that it is uniquely experienced by each individual.

However, it is equally the case that there are clear similarities between people who are suffering. First, they show high levels of distress in relation to their physical or mental anguish. Second, suffering individuals give negative meanings to the situations in which they find themselves. These negative meanings may be influenced by the need to guard against the socially stigmatising effects of living with visible or invisible chronic physical conditions or mental health difficulties. In terms of the shared features of suffering, two key words (**loss** and **control**) are particularly important to the experience:

> *According to the authors of the literature examined, the meaning that characterises suffering is quite profound, involving a tremendous sense of the loss of the person's integrity, autonomy, or control over his or her situation or life . . . In suffering, individuals can be thought of as being in the process of losing their very 'humanity', and all the things that are considered to be related to humanness and dignity.*
> (Rodgers and Cowles, 1997, p1050)

Activity 1.4   *Reflection*

Based on your observation of a suffering patient and your own response to this suffering:

- What could be inferred about how the individual experienced suffering?
- On what grounds did you make this inference?
- What communication/interpersonal interventions were helpful/would be helpful/were needed?

Hint: As with the previous activity, this activity will help you in the development of empathy for suffering human beings.

Healthy relating

From the chapter so far, we can make the following summary statements: good CIPS in nursing are respectful, non-exploitative, non-judgemental and not tainted by everyday casualness. They must be based on the careful development of sensitive helping-trusting relationships with individuals who are suffering. This is because of their perceived loss, and loss of control, of functions, abilities and other attributes that make them human and give them dignity.

However, the above picture of the basis in nursing theory for good, effective and safe CIPS can be broadened with reference to the NMC *Standards for Pre-registration Nursing Education* (2010). The health promotion and education roles of nurses and midwives include a focus that goes beyond a narrow disease orientation to address 'healthy relating'. Healthy relating, in turn, has a developmental basis, a moral basis, a psychological basis and an organisational basis. We will move on to examine each of these now.

The developmental basis for healthy relating

According to Bowlby (1988), relationships between adults mirror the kinds of 'attachment' relationships that can occur between infants and their primary caregivers. In Bowlby's terms, healthy relational living can be described as a series of excursions from a secure base. In **unhealthy relating**, individuals avoid such excursions for fear of abandonment or the removal of their secure base.

There are clear implications emerging from such 'healthy' and 'unhealthy' attachment styles for interpersonal communication between nurses and midwives and their patients or clients. Arguably, the most important of these is that patients may need to be helped to feel reasonably secure in their relationship with nurses. This is achieved through nurses offering their patients/clients time, within which they listen non-judgementally to those they care for. From the perspective of secure relationships, more healthily attached individuals, who feel listened to, understood and supported, will be more able to take risks towards independent living and increased health.

Activity 1.5 — *Team working*

- With your peers, think of children you knew when you were very young. Can you distinguish between those who were timid and shy and those who were very confident 'natural leaders'? How might their respective home and parental environments have contributed to their shyness and confidence?
- Think of people you know currently. Can you distinguish between 'non-risk takers' and 'risk takers'? Is there anything about the early lives of each group that may have contributed to their current respective styles around risk?
- Apply the above two scenario questions to yourself, and consider your answers in relation to your own levels of confidence and risk-taking style. Identify people in your family or among your friends who either inhibit or encourage your confidence and risk taking.
- Now, apply the two scenario questions to patients you know. What kinds of relationships with healthcare staff might help patients feel enabled to take risks towards independent living and increased health?

Hint: This activity will hopefully help you develop greater sensitivity and understanding towards the difficulties patients/clients have in working towards independent living, and your awareness of yourself in this regard.

The moral basis for healthy relating

The provision of time to be listened to, by nurses and midwives, may be something of a novelty for some people in receipt of nursing care. One reason for this is that they have gone through their lives being treated as objects in various ways. This could include being treated as a precious object who must not be damaged in any way, an unwanted object whose presence is a constant nuisance, or a useless object who can do nothing right.

The work of the philosopher Martin Buber (1958) is helpful in understanding the ethical basis for healthy relationships. In simplified form, Buber's argument is that we all have a choice to relate to each other either as objects (what he terms 'I–it' relationships) or as full human beings ('I–thou' relationships). Full human relating amounts to the ethical practice of respectful attention to, and respect for, the inner world, feelings, beliefs and viewpoints of the other person.

Using Buber's terminology, the experience of being treated as an 'I' rather than an 'it' is more likely to lead to individuals feeling self-confident and independent, and trusting of their own worth, judgement and feelings. This in turn may well help them to begin to develop more healthy relationships, both with themselves, in terms of having greater **self-esteem**, and with others.

Theory summary: Self-esteem

Self-esteem reflects the emotions that result from individuals' appraisal of their overall effectiveness in the conduct of their lives (Hewitt, 1998). Self-esteem is thus clearly subjective and develops from individuals' perceptions of themselves and their achievements. This is particularly so in interpersonal relationships and relates to the value and significance we place on our views of ourselves – or our self-concept.

To complicate matters, a person may have many objective achievements and still have low self-esteem. Conversely, individuals with few achievements who believe they have conducted themselves as well as they could in life can have high self-esteem. In healthcare, patients, clients or service users often experience a lowering of self-esteem because they are unable to function as they would normally. They might previously have had satisfactory levels of self-esteem or an ability to aspire to achieve higher levels.

Yet levels of self-esteem can be maintained throughout periods of ill health if patients are given appropriate levels of support. This works in two ways: either individuals' health creates such a threat to their self-identity that they become emotionally immobilised, or they will be sufficiently challenged by the illness or change in health that they develop new coping skills that result in an increase in self-esteem. The nurse's role is to provide support and confirmation of the person's efforts to help protect the individual's self-esteem.

The psychological basis for healthy relating

Some individuals who have experienced a lifetime of being mistreated, and who therefore regard themselves in Buber's terms as an 'it', have from a very young age had their inner world of meanings and feelings constantly disregarded by those who have been in the closest contact with them. Those in closest contact with young children are normally their parents and, a little later, their teachers and peers at school. The influence of these close contacts can have a considerable effect on a person's psychological well-being and sense of self-esteem and self-worth. These ideas and interpretations of the meanings of experiences with others form the basis of an individual's own theory of the reasons for things happening the way they do around or to him or her. This is known as the **theory of mind** and plays a large part in influencing the psychological basis for healthy relating to others.

Theory summary: Theory of mind

In a dynamic interactive way, human beings make constant judgements about each other. The 'theory of mind' concept is implicated in social and emotional intelligence (Goleman, 2006; Smith and Grant, 2014) and is linked to the development of compassionate sensibilities (Gilbert, 2009). It refers to how we all make more or less intelligent inferences and guesses about what we think are the causes of each other's behaviours, and what is going through each other's minds, based on our levels of neuropsychological development (Baron-Cohen, 2003; Goleman, 2006).

The human ability to have a theory of mind seems to be important for us in order to 'read' and respond to interpersonal situations well enough to get by relatively smoothly, helpfully and with some degree of compassion for others on a day-to-day basis. However, theory of mind is a specific skill and some people vary in their levels of emotional and cognitive attunement with others. At one extreme, individuals described either as psychopathic (Howe, 2013) or as having an antisocial personality disorder (Davidson et al., 2010) have neither the developed abilities for emotional, empathic and cognitive connection with others nor concern about this.

Others experience difficulties in being able to guess what is going on in other people's minds or read their emotions, because of their experience of poor parenting as children. In this group of people, the fact that their emotions were constantly invalidated by the adults in their lives may result in them having retarded neuropsychological development to the extent that they lack functional compassion for themselves, and thus with others (Arntz and Van Gerderen, 2009; Gilbert, 2009; Grant, 2010b; Howe, 2013). Sometimes, as in the case of how young children are (mis)treated by their parents and/or teachers, it is sadly the case that what's going on in the minds of the former is of little importance to the latter.

The work of Baron-Cohen (2003), although in large part dealing with Asperger's syndrome, has wider implications for the psychological basis of healthy relating (Goleman, 2006). As with the ability to be empathic, described below, people in general differ in their ability to judge accurately the internal world of another, and this truism applies to nurses as much as it does to any other group of people. This has clear implications for the ongoing development of skilled interpersonal communication in nursing. Nursing students should not assume that they are highly skilled in this area, and may have to work hard at developing this ability (Goleman, 2006).

Empathy

Developing empathic sensibilities

The first scenario on page 9 above, of Jenny, a first-year student nurse responding to a patient's distress, illustrates the privileging of what Goffman (1959) described as *impression management* over empathic responding. Impression management refers to the priority given to the need to demonstrate and develop a positive identity in social contexts where we want to enhance our sense of belonging to a specific social group, in line with social identity theory (Tajfel, 1982) and self-categorisation theory (Turner et al., 1987).

In the short term, acting on such a need may well provide Jenny with the sense of value, worth and belonging she requires from her qualified nursing colleagues. However, in so doing Jenny is equally making a clear statement about the status of the groups that are *othered* (Canales, 2000). In her case, these are the patients who are supposedly in her 'care' and their relatives, who are, by dint of her actions, treated as having less worth, social status and value compared with her professional reference group. Jenny is also acting as her own role model in replicating longstanding power and communication imbalances, described throughout this text as characteristic of poor interpersonal nursing. She is laying down a template for her own future style of non-responsiveness to patients' interpersonal needs.

The strong emphasis of this book on compassionate CIPS requires undergraduate student nurses to behave more like Susan than Jenny, in managing the construction of a social identity which gives equal respect and credence to anti-othering practices and the *humanising* of healthcare as well as the need to be liked and valued by one's colleagues. The need to develop *empathic sensibilities* involves role taking: putting yourself in the place of another person and imagining what it might be like for them to be in that situation. This links both to compassionate practice and the performance of non-visible psychological care (Bach, 2004), and to the idea from self-categorisation theory that the perception of people as similar to you makes an empathic response from you more likely. This is because you will more readily identify with their pain, on the basis that 'an injury to them is an injury to me' (Levine and Crowther, 2008; Drury et al., 2009). However, on the basis of both social identity and self-categorisation theories, it is worth emphasising that how each student nurse considers the social identity of what it means to be a nurse will influence their actions. For example, Jenny could believe that not interrupting the task she has been given, to respond to patient distress, corresponds to the nursing social identity she aspires to – that of the task-focused nurse. Conversely, Susan may see the social identity of nurses as being *always* about compassion and the unconditional alleviation of distress.

Responding to how patients and clients perceive their life-worlds necessitates the development of empathic sensibilities among nursing students. Linking to Activity 1.4 above, developing empathic sensibilities is fundamental to the broader requirement for nursing students to hone their critical thinking, and requires the increasing honing of the *empathic imagination* life skill. Because the range of possible life-worlds that people occupy is vast in our plural, postmodern and multicultural societies, it's a tall order to expect students and qualified nurses to be empathically geared up to every variant of possible human suffering they may possibly come into contact with. However, you can develop your empathic sensibilities by the regular exercise of empathic imagination. This can be achieved by either engaging with films and books which emphasise the importance of sensitively stepping into the shoes of another, or by reading narratives from people whose lives have been compromised by serious and often tragic interruptions (discussed in Chapter 2).

Activity 1.6   *Developing an empathic imagination*

Below are two possibilities for honing your empathic imagination:

1. Check out the fictional psychological profiler, Dr Tony Hill, in the novels of crime writer, Val McDermid (www.valmcdermid.com). In these novels, and in the television series *Wire in the Blood* which is based on them, McDermid skilfully and intelligently explores the relationship between people, such as the central character Tony Hill, who have highly developed empathy skills, and psychopathic criminals, who are grossly deficient in this area. Explore the ways in which Hill's empathic sophistication, and the empathy deficits of the people he helps bring to justice, are in both cases related to their respective upbringings. What lessons can you learn from McDermid's work about how you can develop your own empathic imagination?
2. The *Our Encounters* series of books contains narratives from people who have experienced health-related problems and treatment characterised by poor and unhelpful communication at the hands of health practitioners, including nurses. Try to step into the shoes of these people by reading stories from *Our Encounters with Madness* (Grant et al., 2011), *Our Encounters with Suicide* (Grant et al., 2013) or *Our Encounters with Self-Harm* (Baker et al., 2013). Identify the surprises you experience while reading these stories, and how they made you feel.

Empathy defined

According to Howe (2013), the word 'empathy' entered the English language in the early years of the twentieth century. Its roots are in the Greek word *empatheia*, which means *to enter feelings from the outside, or to be with a person's feelings, passions or suffering* (Howe, 2013, p9). The capacity to do this is clearly fundamental to understanding, interpreting and compassionately locating meaning in people and their situations, thus to be successful in human-to-human relating. It is captured succinctly in the shorter definition, provided by Kohut (1984), who described empathy as the capacity to think and feel oneself into the inner life of another person.

From a more specialised psychotherapeutic standpoint, which however captures the need for nurses to be able to *demonstrate* empathy to and with the people in their care, Rogers defined empathy as occurring when:

the therapist is sensing the feelings and personal meanings which the client is experiencing
in each moment, when he [sic] *can perceive these from 'inside', as they seem to the client, and*
when he can successfully communicate something of that understanding to his client.
(Rogers, 1967, p62)

Given the importance that theory of mind plays in the psychological basis for healthy relating generally, as discussed above, it seems difficult to argue against the importance for nursing of the ability to enter another person's feelings and, without losing necessary objectivity, see the world through that person's eyes and demonstrate this. However, on the basis of the cumulative evidence from the literature, Lauder et al. (2002) argued that many recipients of healthcare professional interventions, including nursing care, do not believe that professionals understand either their feelings or their perspectives. In addition to constituting a fundamental violation of compassionate interpersonal relating, it is clear that a limited ability to identify and understand the feelings and perspectives of people in their care may result in such care being substandard. This will fail to meet the goals and needs of patients and their relatives and/or carers, in preventing these groups from having a collaborative and inclusive role in both problem solving and achieving optimal health outcomes (Tait, 1985; Sloane, 1993).

Empathy in context

There are two important contexts for the exercise of empathy: the interpersonal context and, in related and broader terms, the organisational context.

The interpersonal context

Greenberg (2007) argues that health workers who display empathy both enable patients and clients to become self-soothing and are more likely to create a good emotional relationship with them. In short, the health worker who conveys genuine interest, acceptance, caring, compassion and joy, and no anger, contempt, disgust or fear, creates the environment for a secure emotional bond. On the basis of this argument, nurses' facial, postural and vocal expressions of emotion clearly have the potential to set very different emotional climates. Based on evidence from neuroscience, Greenberg argues that patients'/clients' right-brain hemispheres respond more to nurses' facial communication than to nurses' words. Quite simply, patients/clients learn who they are, and how acceptable they are, from the facial expressions of their nurses, irrespective of what nurses actually say to them. Frequently, nurses may 'say the right things' to patients/clients, their relatives and carers, only for their facial expressions to contradict their words, while simultaneously lacking any awareness of the contradiction occurring between the two modes of communication. The net result of this is that they may at best appear shallow, patronising and/or insensitive, and at worst downright dishonest.

Case study: Avoiding anger

John is a nursing student in his first year. He was a sensitive, quiet child, and one of a large family, in a volatile, sometimes violent, household. He is uncomfortable with patients expressing their anger in his presence, and frequently feels disgust towards such patients. He would far rather avoid such anger, so he begins to act out a pattern of being available only for happy patients. He is not sufficiently aware of this to acknowledge it or to do anything about it. This pattern will go largely unnoticed by qualified staff and will continue after he qualifies as a registered nurse.

In addition to understanding the complexity of an individual's personal theory of mind and its impact on CIPS, being empathic requires the ability not just to think about the mind of the other but to respond to that person's emotional state accurately (Goleman, 2006; Greenberg, 2007). Empathy can therefore be described as the ability to be intuitively aware of what another person is feeling as well as thinking.

Being able to perceive, understand and respond appropriately to another person's emotions is not easy. This is because people can hide or disguise their emotions with behaviours that can contradict how they actually feel. We learn how to communicate our understanding of another's feelings through verbal and non-verbal expressions and then (here comes the tricky bit) interpret those signals accurately. In healthcare, this complex interaction takes place in settings that are often far from ideal – for example, on busy wards, being overheard by others, during painful experiences or on hearing bad news.

In these situations, nurses and midwives have to draw upon their professional inner resources to try to feel the emotions their patient feels, while at the same time maintaining a separate identity. It is important to recognise which feelings belong to the patient and which to the nurse. This is a difficult skill to learn and Chapter 3 will provide more guidance on how to develop this ability.

Trust and respect

Other theoretical concepts to consider when judging and engaging with patients in relation to empathy are *trust* and *respect*. Trust is based upon our previous experiences and enables individuals to cope with the world and resolve frustrations about those things that may be unfamiliar or unknown. Respect, in turn contingent on honesty, consistency, faith and hope, is an element of a trusting relationship. Once these elements are established, a sharing of emotions and thoughts can take place.

Empathic attunement

Complementing Benner's views on 'emotional attunement' (discussed in the introduction to this chapter) is Greenberg's (2007) concept of 'empathic attunement' (see also Howe, 2013). Derived from scientific research, empathic attunement suggests that nurses and midwives who convey genuine interest, acceptance and caring are more likely to achieve a secure emotional bond with their patients. In this regard, as argued above, non-verbal facial communication is extremely important. Essentially, patients/clients learn how acceptable they are from the facial expressions of healthcare staff.

Case study: Reacting to a patient's story

While sitting by the bedside of one of her patients, a first-year student adult nurse hears a story from the patient's past that makes her feel disturbed and somewhat disgusted. The patient has disclosed that, when she was in her early teens, she had a sexual relationship with her brother, which may or may not have been entirely consensual. Mindful of the importance of facial expression in empathic communication, the nurse makes an effort to match her supportive and sensitive response to the patient's disclosure with a facial expression that signifies care and concern rather than shock and disgust.

What do you think she should say to the patient, and how best should she say it so that her words reasonably cohere with her facial expression, being mindful of the fact that she feels she needs to balance honesty with compassion and non-judgementalism?

The organisational basis for healthy relating

The discussion so far has hopefully illustrated the importance of nurses and midwives working towards secure rather than insecure attachment styles with their patients/clients, and supporting them in a health-promoting way to believe more in themselves, and in their emotions and judgements. However, the above bases for healthy relationships, and the skilled practice of CIPS, depend in turn upon healthy and health-promoting work settings.

Contemporary nurses need to be able to engage in problem solving, critical thinking and reflection around safe and effective CIPS within the complex and varied care environments that characterise health provision in the twenty-first century. These behaviours should be carried out in the context of multidisciplinary practice, and be fair, professionally and ethically appropriate, as well as responsive to the needs of diverse patient populations.

Environments shape experience

Sadly, the nature and influence of healthcare organisations is a much neglected area in nursing and health CIPS books. This is surprising, given the strong message emerging from the social psychological literature that organisational social environments play a part in shaping experience and identity (Tajfel, 1982; Turner et al., 1987; Meyerson, 2002; Zimbardo, 2009) at both conscious (rational) and unconscious (including irrational) levels (Morgan, 2006; Alvesson and Spicer, 2012).

> ### Concept summary: External and internal environments
>
> By external environment, we mean all the features that seem external to patients/clients and staff, and that can have an influence on their perception, experience of, reaction to, and involvement in healthcare. These features include inpatient or outpatient healthcare environments, such as wards or clinics, and staff and patient cultures.
>
> Patients' internal environmental state is derived from their physiological, spiritual, psychological, developmental and social characteristics. These internal states will have been influenced by beliefs from family, friends or the media, and by any previous experiences they have had of healthcare settings.

Two views of healthcare organisations

Organisational social science suggests that work organisations can be thought about and experienced on a spectrum made up of both irrational and rational features, and that every organisation contains both of these features in different ways (Alvesson and Spicer, 2012). However, at a common-sense level, we often experience the healthcare organisations within which we undertake our practice placements as simply the settings where people work together to carry out the delivery of high-quality nursing care. Positioned squarely in the rational area of the spectrum, this implicit view of organisations suggests that they can be always trusted as constituting reasonable and well-intentioned places to work in. From a rational perspective, the work of the people in the organisation is regarded as separate from the organisation itself or from what people think about the organisation.

However, an entirely different picture of healthcare organisations is possible, sometimes referred to as the 'social constructionist' view of organisations. From a social constructionist perspective, the process of thinking and acting together within specific organisational circumstances contributes over time to a social and cultural agreement about 'the way things are done here'. The socially constructed organisation is simultaneously rational and irrational (Pfeffer, 1981; Grant, 2000; Grant and Townend, 2007; Morgan, 2006; Alvesson and Spicer, 2012).

The social constructionist view of organisations shifts the focus away from simple 'bricks and mortar' assumptions of what organisations are about. From a rational perspective, organisations are simply physical structures within which employees work. From a rational and irrational-social constructionist perspective, organisations are social psychological structures that individuals create together in their day-to-day interactions.

When considered in the context of healthcare organisations that function both rationally and irrationally simultaneously, we should not be surprised by the unfortunate fact, reported by many patients/clients and often confirmed by staff, that 'the way things are done' in some work settings is clearly to the disadvantage of the communication and interpersonal needs of patients/clients. This is illustrated in the following case study.

> **Case study: A negative culture**
>
> *A student nurse is on a practice learning experience in a nursing home that cares for often immobile, elderly clients. He notices that the qualified nurses and assistant nurses often don't speak to their clients as they give them bed baths and feed them. This seems to be part of the 'culture' of the home. Residents are treated as if they are objects rather than human beings, and the nurses seem more interested in their lives outside work. Little or no attention is paid to the esteem needs of the residents who are left to a lonely, monochrome and unstimulating existence rather than a life.*

Task versus person orientation

In clear violation of the ethic of healthy relating, in the senses discussed above, sometimes patients are treated as objects rather than people. This is because the work culture is task- rather than person-oriented, in spite of such things as glossy, locally produced mission statements to the contrary, or on the welcoming name boards outside rest homes and nursing homes. According to the research and theorising of Menzies Lyth (1988), nursing task-orientation functions as a social system to defend against anxiety. From this perspective, it is arguably less demanding, or anxiety provoking, to treat patients or clients as 'bodies' to be washed, fed or dressed, rather than as people to be listened to, or to be involved in their care and in healthcare decisions made about them. According to Menzies Lyth, the degree of intimacy that might come with person-oriented care is perceived at an individual- and organisational-unconscious level to bring with it the danger of being overwhelmed by sharing in the suffering of patients.

Morgan (2006), another organisational theorist, provides a framework to help us understand the ways in which, at an irrational level, healthcare organisations may unconsciously defend themselves against the guilt that would arise if they honestly admitted that they were task- rather than patient-oriented (a theme to be developed in Chapter 3). Drawing on Freudian principles, Morgan argues that organisations often protect themselves by using *defence mechanisms*. At an individual level, defence mechanisms refer to the ways in which individuals maintain an acceptable social face by defending themselves against blame and guilt, in a way that is outside their awareness. Morgan argues that this process can occur on a larger scale, at the level of the socially constructed organisation. A common organisational defence mechanism is **rationalisation**. In the context of day-to-day nursing work, rationalisation might be seen to occur when nurses give plausible reasons for not spending time with their clients and listening to their concerns. 'Too busy' or 'not enough time' are often given as rationalised reasons. However, if tasks rather than people denote a deeply engrained work culture, having more time is unlikely to change these cultural practices.

Busyness affecting group and individual behaviour

A 'we're too busy' stance might contain more than a grain of truth in circumstances where there are staff shortages. However, as discussed above, a basic understanding of the ways in which nurses and other healthcare staff think and behave in groups, in relation to how they identify with, and behave in them at conscious and less than conscious levels, may add to our understanding of the social psychological, organisational processes whereby clients' communication and interpersonal needs are either often ignored or treated as an irritant. This may especially be the case if these needs are seen by staff to conflict with the real business of the healthcare setting.

Patients who seek attention from nursing staff, often for very good reasons, may be negatively 'labelled' in these circumstances. This type of mindset, frequently observable in a range of nursing work groups, is defensive and, complementary to Menzies Lyth's and Morgan's theorising, usually serves an anxiety reduction function. If challenged about it, nurses would very likely deny any wrongdoing on their part and would probably give a rationalised answer.

Thus, mindsets may take the form of 'them and us' thinking, where 'us' is viewed as reasonable and hardworking and 'them' as manipulative and troublesome. Unfortunately, 'them and us' thinking is associated with the production of irrational prejudice (Dixon and Levine, 2012), based on often insufficiently informed first impressions, with a failure to read patients/clients correctly and fairly at either empathic or theory-of-mind levels.

Belonging to the group or standing up for the patient?

In ending this section, we invite student nurses to engage in a challenge. This is to be aware and to recognise when the kinds of healthcare group processes discussed above are happening to the disadvantage of the communication and interpersonal needs of their patients or clients, and to act appropriately. The professional ethics of nursing practice, NMC standards and the need to respond in an emotionally and empathically attuned way to your patient may pull you in one direction, while the need to retain the good opinion of the work group pulls you in the other. At the start of your career, and into the future, how might you resolve this dilemma?

Chapter summary

This chapter has emphasised the importance of student nurses making their own assessment of their CIPS at the start of their pre-registration training programme. The importance of CIPS was contextualised in relation to national and international nursing policy and educational literature. Communication frameworks governing CIPS were discussed and analysed, as was the relationship between CIPS and caring, moral practice, suffering, empathy and healthy relating in nursing.

Further reading

Chambers, C and Ryder, E (2009) *Compassion and Caring in Nursing.* Oxford: Radcliffe Publishing. This book will provide you with a very useful, more indepth exploration of the concepts of compassion and caring.

Frost, PJ, Dutton, JE, Worlen, MC and Wilson, A (2000) Narratives of compassion in organizations. In: Fineman, S (ed.) *Emotion in Organizations*, 2nd edn. London: Sage.

Gilbert, P (2009) *The Compassionate Mind.* London: Constable.

Howe, D (2013) *Empathy: What it is and why it matters.* Basingstoke: Palgrave Macmillan.

The above texts provide a thoroughly evidence-based approach to the development of compassion, and empathy as an integral dimension of compassion. They will help you develop more of an understanding of how nursing and healthcare generally can and should be made more human, as an antidote to cold, heartless and unpleasant healthcare environments.

Drury, J, Cocking, C and Reicher, S (2009) Everyone for themselves? A comparative study of crowd solidarity among emergency survivors. *British Journal of Social Psychology,* 48: 487–506.

Levine, M and Crowther, S (2008) The responsive bystander: how social group membership and group size can encourage as well as inhibit bystander intervention. *Journal of Personality and Social Psychology,* 95(6): 1429–1439.

Tajfel, H (ed.) (1982) *Social Identity Intergroup Relations* (pp15–40). Cambridge: Cambridge University Press.

Turner, JC, Hogg, MA, Oakes, PJ, Reicher, SD and Weatherell, MS (1987) *Rediscovering the Social Group: A social categorisation theory.* Oxford: Blackwell.

This collection of books and articles will help you develop your understanding of the relationship between nursing identity, group membership and responsive action.

Useful websites

www.bbcprisonstudy.org

Two UK social psychologists recreated the Stanford prison experiment for a BBC documentary in 2002. This interactive website explores their findings and the implications for the psychology of groups and how we view power, obedience and resistance.

www.compassionatemind.co.uk

Set up in 2006, The Compassionate Mind Foundation aims to promote well-being through the scientific understanding and application of compassion. We're sure you will enjoy using this excellent website.

www.culturediversity.org/basic.htm

This site introduces you to Leininger's theory of transcultural nursing. This is a humanistic and scientific area of formal study and practice in nursing, which is focused on differences and similarities among cultures with respect to human care, health and illness, based on people's cultural values, beliefs and practices. The intention is to promote the use of this knowledge to provide culture-specific or culturally congruent nursing care to people.

www.dignityincare.org.uk

This is the website for the Dignity in Care network, which aims to end tolerance of indignity in health and social care services by raising awareness and inspiring people to take action.

https://www.gov.uk/government/uploads/system/uploads/attachment_data/file/216695/dh_119973.pdf

This is the link for the Department of Health's *Essence of Care* series, which gives useful guidelines and audit tools that can be downloaded.

www.watsoncaringscience.org/caring_science/index.html

This site introduces you to the theory of caring science and the foundations of Watson's transpersonal theory. The theory was developed to bring meaning and focus to nursing and make explicit nursing's values, knowledge and practices of human caring that are geared towards subjective inner healing processes. It is based on the notion of cherishing.

Chapter 2
Evidence-based communication and interpersonal skills

NMC Standards for Pre-registration Nursing Education

This chapter will address the following competencies:

Domain 2: Communication and interpersonal skills

4. All nurses must recognise when people are anxious or in distress and respond effectively, using therapeutic principles to promote their wellbeing, manage personal safety and resolve conflict. They must use effective communication strategies and negotiation techniques to achieve best outcomes, respecting the dignity and human rights of all concerned. They must know when to consult a third party and how to make referrals for advocacy, mediation or arbitration.

NMC Essential Skills Clusters

This chapter will address the following ESCs:

Cluster: Care, compassion and communication

1. As partners in the care process, people can trust a newly registered graduate nurse to provide collaborative care based on the highest standards, knowledge and competence.

By the first progression point:

3. Promotes a professional image.

By the second progression point:

7. Uses professional support structures to learn from experience and make appropriate adjustments.

Chapter aims

After reading this chapter, you should be able to:

*   outline the evidence base for CIPS in nursing;
*   understand the differences and tensions between narrow and broad readings of 'evidence-based practice';

- understand key issues in the historical development of research in CIPS in nursing;
- understand the relative contribution of counselling and psychotherapy models for the practice of CIPS;
- understand what is meant by patient first- and second-level forms of communication;
- describe some evidence-based principles for the practice of CIPS.

Introduction

This chapter will enable you to analyse and critically evaluate the literature on evidence-based CIPS relevant to nursing practice. First, we will address the question: do CIPS in nursing make a difference? We will then explore the significance of CIPS in the NMC *Standards for Pre-registration Nursing Education*, in relation to both evidence-based nursing practice and evidence-based health-care, from the perspective of narrow and broader readings of what constitutes the evidence base. Following this, the chapter will take a more focused view of the history and development of research in interpersonal communication in nursing. The discussion will then turn to issues around teaching and learning, and the issue of the uptake of skilled interpersonal communication among nurses. You will hopefully see that the nursing literature in this area relatively ignores key research and theoretical work on the importance of the context of interpersonal communication, including the organisational, or work-setting, context. From this basis, you will be able to evaluate the relative contribution of counselling and psychotherapy models of CIPS. We will argue that, while these models claim to provide useful principles for practice, they must be modified according to work-setting contexts. Their usefulness must also be evaluated in the context of contemporary critiques of the humanistic basis for counselling models popular in nursing and theory and research in the area of social cognition – the study of how people process social information (there is more on social cognition, or social thinking, in Chapter 3).

The chapter will end by providing you with a set of evidence-based principles for practice, and we will also include information from conceptual, empirical and policy literature about what it means to be client/patient- and carer-centred.

Do CIPS make a difference?

Backing up ordinary human experience or common sense, both CIPS research (Hargie and Dickson, 2004; Hargie, 2006) and, in a complementary way, psychotherapy research (Norcross, 2002; Gilbert and Leahy, 2007) suggest that there is every reason to accept that the skilful practice of CIPS makes a positive, healing difference to patients. Specifically, this includes them:

- feeling listened to;
- feeling that their concerns are being validated and not trivialised;
- feeling supported;
- feeling understood.

Evidence-based CIPS in nursing practice

The NMC *Standards for Pre-registration Nursing Education* (2010) argue that nursing practice, integrated with theory, needs to be evidence-based, and thus safe. There are good reasons why the safe and effective practice of CIPS in nursing should aim to be evidence-based. With regard to a conventional reading of the meaning of evidence-based nursing, practices are considered safe and effective either because of a developing body of research-based scientific (sometimes called 'empirical') knowledge to support them, or because of theoretical consensus. 'Theoretical consensus' means large-scale agreement, built up over a long time, by communities of nursing practitioners and academics, and scholars from outside the discipline whose work has been seen to have relevance for nursing.

Together, researchers and theorists have contributed to the systematic consideration about, reflection on and refinement of nursing CIPS practice. This contrasts strongly with the notion of simply relating to, and communicating with, patients/clients in particular styles because 'it's always been done that way' or because 'it's quick and easy'. This also points to CIPS in nursing with people having healthcare needs as being distinct from everyday communication between people in general.

The theory summaries that follow will introduce you to key fundamental issues and tensions around both the meaning and principles of evidence-based healthcare practice, and the activities and sections that follow this box will help you begin to engage with some systematically developed theoretical and scientific concerns.

Theory summary: Evidence-based healthcare from a conventional or narrow perspective

Conventional, or hitherto relatively uncontested, understandings of evidence-based healthcare privilege quantitative-experimental research that demonstrates statistically significant, proven outcomes of experiments. These experiments systematically test out interventions for health problems against control group interventions, to see if the former actually result in health benefits. To strengthen confidence in the results of individual experiments that do demonstrate such benefits, systematic reviews of groups of them are subject to further statistical analysis. This further increases confidence in specific interventions over others. However, research alone is not the only factor in judging the worth of evidence from a conventional perspective. The work of Muir Gray (1997), Trinder and Reynolds (2000) and Sackett et al. (2004) is seminal in representing the view that healthcare practice should be based on the combination of three factors. These are:

- the best available evidence;
- the values of society;
- the resources available.

These authors argue that the practice of evidence-based healthcare based on conventional understandings of its meaning is conducted on the basis of an established hierarchy of strength of evidence, described below, where 1 is assumed to be the source of evidence that healthcare practitioners can have most confidence in.

1. strong evidence from at least one systematic review of multiple and well-designed randomised control trials;

2. strong evidence from at least one properly designed randomised control trial of an appropriate size;

3. evidence from well-designed research trials that do not contain randomisation, for example single-group, pre–post, cohort, time series or matched case-control studies;

4. evidence from well-designed, non-experimental studies from more than one centre or research group;

5. opinions of respected authorities, based on clinical evidence, descriptive studies, reports or expert committees.

Evidence-based healthcare from a broader perspective

While acknowledging the worth of the above model of evidence-based healthcare and its obvious benefits, recent years have seen a growing critique of the above assumptions, principles and related practices as the *sole* basis for understanding the meaning, practice and extent of evidence-based healthcare. This is because of the argument that the conventional model exclusively derives from and reinforces biomedical understandings of both 'health' and 'recovery', suppresses other forms of understandings and fails to live up to its claims of neutrality and objectivity (Zeeman et al., 2014a, b).

Alternative forms of knowledge, such as service user and practitioner narratives, sometimes described as knowledge from the 'lived experience' paradigm (world-view), yield equally valid but different types of information (Grant et al., 2011, 2013; Baker, 2013; Grant, 2014a; Grant and Leigh-Phippard, 2014). While randomised control trials tell us important things about *outcomes* of experiments on various interventions in health research, they are less concerned with the various ways in which patients and clients *experience* such interventions. To be concerned only with the former at the expense of the latter gives an incomplete, one-dimensional picture of evidence-based healthcare and what it can offer.

For example, with great relevance for CIPS in nursing and healthcare more generally, Charon (2001) argues that *narrative competence*, or the *competence that human beings use to absorb, interpret, and respond to stories*, facilitates empathic, professional and trustworthy practice. In a complementary way, Greenhalgh and Hurwitz (1999) assert that attention to patients' narratives facilitates methods for addressing existential qualities such as inner hurt, despair, hope, grief and moral pain, which both frequently accompany, and sometimes constitute, the health problems that people experience. Both Charon and Greenhalgh and Hurwitz argue that narratives of illness provide a framework for approaching a patient's problems holistically and for identifying diagnostic and therapeutic options. *Writing for Recovery*, for example – a recent therapeutic development in mental health – is a framework for helping people enhance their mental health recovery through helping them engage in creative writing about their experiences (Taylor et al., 2014).

Activity 2.1   *Team working*

The meaning of evidence-based healthcare in practice

With a group of fellow students, identify the possible ways in which qualified nurses and other healthcare practitioners might respond to a group discussion of the two different readings of evidence-based healthcare outlined above.

Hint: This activity will prepare you for being able to engage intelligently and in an informed way with future discussions in practice.

You will find possible answers to this activity at the end of the chapter.

The historical development of research in CIPS in nursing

The historical development of an evidence-based interest in CIPS in nursing is well documented. According to MacLeod Clark (1985), research interest in the area developed throughout the latter half of the twentieth century and included patient satisfaction surveys; studies exploring the benefits of improved communication; observational studies that described and analysed the ways in which nurses and their patients/clients interacted; and studies on the effectiveness of interpersonal skills teaching.

Banister and Kagan (1985) argued that research work on interpersonal skills in nursing was influenced by research traditions in other fields, including sociology, counselling, and social, clinical and management psychology. From these disciplines, a set of desirable skills emerged, particularly social skills, empathy and assertiveness.

Thus, during the latter decades of the twentieth century, nursing interpersonal research was greatly influenced by social skills and assertion training assumptions (Davidson, 1985). It was assumed that, in order to develop and hone interpersonal skills, nurses and their patients/clients needed to be both socially skilled and assertive. This is indicated by the circular view that the interpersonally skilled nurse is defined as such by having social and assertiveness skills (and group facilitation skills) (Morrison and Burnard, 1991).

Activity 2.2   *Evidence-based practice and research*

With a group of fellow students, consider what the range of challenges might be with regard to implementing evidence-based CIPS in the work settings you've come across in your practice learning experiences.

Hint: This activity will help develop your awareness that the transfer of evidence-based CIPS to organisational practice is not a straightforward matter.

You will find possible answers to this activity at the end of the chapter.

The relationship between research in CIPS and teaching, experiential learning and organisational practice

The above nursing interpersonal research, in turn, influenced assumptions around developing a 'lifelong learning' approach to acquiring interpersonal skills as a feature of professional development and **experiential learning**:

> *The most obvious methods of monitoring progress in interpersonal skills development [are] . . . practising the skills involved and . . . noticing our changing and developing reactions. The practice element often comes with the job. We are involved in interpersonal relationships every day of our professional lives so there is plenty of time for trying out new behaviour. It has to be noted, however, that the decision to try out new interpersonal behaviour must be a conscious one. It is very easy to attend a workshop on counselling skills and to believe that a lot was gained from it. The truth is of course that the workshop will only have been successful if the learning gained in it is transferred to the 'real' situation. There is always a danger of an interpersonal skills workshop being an 'island' in the middle of a busy working life – something that was interesting at the time, but of little practical value.* (Burnard, 1996, p93)

Activity 2.3   *Team working*

A group of busy nurses go on a communication course and learn the principles of good CIPS. They return to their ward and, after a month, the ward manager wonders why the number of complaints about poor communication hasn't gone down at all. Discuss as a group why this might be.

Brown et al. (2006) critiqued the standpoint that a communication skill, once learned, can be readily transferred from one context to another. In particular, these authors challenged a central assumption displayed by nurse scholars such as Burnard and others. This is that the kind of communication skills deriving from counselling models, which by definition depend on dedicated communication time, can reasonably be transferred to busier contexts where there is very little time available.

Activity 2.4   *Reflection*

Think about the various contexts within which you try to communicate effectively with your clients. What are the contextual factors that both facilitate and limit good communication?

Hint: Contexts may be personal, interpersonal or environmental.

An apparent lack of attention to the ways in which organisational contextual factors may undermine the practice of skilled interpersonal communication is displayed in much of the writing on CIPS in nursing. This phenomenon may be linked to continual frustration about the fact that, although skilled interpersonal communication is talked up in nurse education and literature, its practice in real-life healthcare situations leaves a lot to be desired (MacLeod Clark, 1985). Brown et al. (2006) argued that this is not really surprising, since there are clear contextual differences between what is taught and what is practised:

> *While practitioners may well have absorbed the professional wisdom about the importance of communication in ensuring good outcomes for clients and themselves, they may well continue using timeworn communicative strategies of the kind that lead to complaints, poor outcomes and a sense of alienation between client and practitioner.*
> (Brown et al., 2006, p4)

The Hargie–Dickson model of interpersonal communication and its relevance for nursing

In contrast to literature on interpersonal communication by nurse academics, Hargie and Dickson (2004), who come from a communications rather than a nursing background, were very clear about the major role of contextual factors. Summarising and synthesising research, theory and practice in the area, these authors argued that skilled interpersonal communication can be accounted for in terms of the person–situation context. This means that all communication is context-bound, in that it is always embedded in time, place, the specific form of the relationship of the communicators, and the organisational frameworks within which communication takes place. The personal characteristics of the communicators, together with the above features of the shared situation, act to shape the interaction by determining the goals pursued, and the responses, feedback and perception of the communication event among all those involved. Therefore, if nursing research and teaching on interpersonal communication takes greater account of contextual factors, this may lead to improved CIPS. This may require a shift away from writing, practice and related assumptions about the exclusive relevance of counselling and psychotherapy models of CIPS.

Counselling and psychotherapy models of CIPS and their use in nursing

Despite the concern expressed by Brown and his colleagues about the limitations of counselling and psychotherapy models for the practice of skilled interpersonal communication, a look through the literature on CIPS relevant to nursing reveals a central assumption about the relevance of classic models of counselling and psychotherapy for nursing practice (see, for example, Kagan et al., 1986; Burnard, 1996; Brown et al., 2006; McCabe and Timmins, 2006, 2013). In recent decades, this assumption has resulted in the circular argument that the interpersonally skilled nurse is one who has counselling skills (Morrison and Burnard, 1991).

Clearly, counselling and psychotherapy models have contributed greatly and have transformed nursing theory, knowledge and practice from the mid-twentieth century to date. The work of Carl Rogers (1961), for example, has influenced the shift from a task- to a person-centred and holistic view of nursing care, with specific regard to the adoption of Rogers' 'core conditions' approach to human relating (now known as the 'Rogerian' approach). Rogers identified what he claimed were three *necessary and sufficient* conditions for helping someone change effectively through a good therapeutic relationship. These are:

- acceptance or unconditional positive regard by the nurse for the patient;
- the nurse's therapeutic genuineness;
- empathy.

The Rogerian approach claims its legitimacy on theoretical grounds and on the basis of the respect accorded to it as a therapeutic tradition since the mid-1970s. In marked contrast, cognitive behavioural psychotherapy has always had a robust and impressive evidence base to support its development. It has also brought major benefits to basic and post-basic mental health nursing practice (Grant et al., 2004, 2008, 2010; Grant, 2010a). Since the early 1970s, specialist nurse cognitive behavioural psychotherapists have made a major contribution to the developing theory and practice of both mental health nursing generally (Newell and Gournay, 2000) and cognitive behavioural psychotherapy specifically (Newell and Gournay, 2000; Grant et al., 2004, 2008, 2010).

Cognitive behavioural approaches are increasingly adopting an integrative stance (Gilbert and Leahy, 2007; Grant et al., 2008, 2010). In simple terms, this means that major theoretical and empirical developments from other paradigms are being incorporated into them. One such empirical development, having theoretical roots in psychoanalytic psychotherapy and clear relevance for nursing practices, is the concept of 'transference'.

Theory summary: Transference

Psychotherapy theories have long suggested that the mental representations an individual holds about significant others may either facilitate or impede an individual's progress towards recovery. Significant others are individuals that we have either loved or loathed in our earlier life. A new person can be experienced and treated as either a friend or foe in a matter of moments, a process that largely occurs unconsciously (see Chapter 3). In support of psychotherapy theories, and in line with contemporary developments in social cognition research, Miranda and Andersen (2007) argue that transference occurs automatically in everyday life, when representations of significant others are triggered. Transference is thus a process by which people re-experience past relationships in their everyday social relationships and interactions.

Mental representations of significant others exist in memory, and such representations can easily be triggered by relevant cues in any context. Our global views about ourselves and about significant others are linked in memory. Concurrent activation occurs: when one is activated, the other is too. Transference includes assumptions about the other's presumed feelings about ourself and vice versa, and is directly linked to the concepts of schema, prejudice and stereotyping (see later discussion in this chapter and also Chapter 6).

Evaluating counselling and psychotherapy models for interpersonal communication in nursing

In spite of their benefits, the relevance of some counselling and psychotherapeutic principles for day-to-day nursing care has been criticised from several perspectives. Nurses are charged with the ability to be able to demonstrate cultural and political awareness of their societal role and related professional behaviours (see Chapter 6). In this context, Grant (2002) has highlighted cultural and political concerns with the appropriateness of the **humanistic approach** in general. He encourages students to engage with the literature and debate the role that individualistic psychology, which focuses on the individual without considering societal influences such as politics and paternalism (for example, the 'nanny state'), plays in everyday healthcare practice.

In a comparison of the Rogerian approach with the view of humans as rational (individualistic) economic beings, Howard (2001) argued that Rogerian counsellors concentrate on humans as childlike beings who are not influenced by, or constrained by, the realities of the society in which they live. This society is individualistic, rather than wishing to serve the best interests of all humanity, and is constrained by materialism and 'survival of the fittest'. In this context, Howard proposed that humanistic approaches are naive.

The main criticism to emerge is that we should be wary of a simplistic understanding and practice of **Rogerian principles**. If interpersonal communication is practised independently of the contexts that shape such communication, the differences in organisational power and status between communicators are overlooked.

Further specific criticisms of the relevance of Rogers' core conditions, and related concepts, for nursing practice include challenging the following assumptions:

- that the core conditions are indeed both necessary and sufficient;
- that non-judgementalism is indeed possible between people who are communicating;
- that self-awareness and empathic communication are practised successfully.

These assumptions will be scrutinised, in turn, below.

The core conditions: necessary and sufficient?

From an evidence-based psychotherapeutic perspective, it has long been recognised that, while there is agreement that the core conditions are necessary for good psychotherapeutic relationships, they are often not, in and of themselves, sufficient to help clients with mental health difficulties make changes in themselves and in their lives (see, for example, Beck et al., 1979; Thwaites and Bennett-Levy, 2007). Perhaps at this point it is important to flag up the distinction made earlier between the formal practice of counselling and psychotherapy, and the relevance of using principles deriving from them in the service of developing effective relationships with patients/clients.

Non-judgementalism

There is a crucial question that must be asked by nurses interested in the use of Rogerian core conditions for enhancing CIPS. This is: to what extent is the exercise of non-judgementalism relevant and possible in nursing practice? Based on Rogers' condition of acceptance or unconditional positive regard, humanistic practitioners and writers often advocate non-judgementalism. Burnard, for example, urges health professionals to *try suspending judgement on other people until you fully hear what they say. Even then, try to remain non-judgemental! This skill is one of the basic pre-requisites of effective counselling* (1996, p14).

A major problem with this standpoint is that empirical work in social cognition (social thinking) suggests that it is impossible for human beings to be non-judgemental. It seems necessary, and often helpful for all of us, to take 'cognitive shortcut' judgements to make sense of contextual situations and individuals within those (Augoustinos et al., 2014). As we grow up, we develop what are described as **schemas** to make sense of the world (see Chapter 6). Schemas can be thought of as mental structures that contain broad expectations and knowledge of the world. These are more or less adaptive in regard to how they prepare us to engage with people and events in our lives, and include general expectations about people, social roles, social events and how to behave in specific situations (Hargie and Dickson, 2004; Grant, 2010b; Grant et al., 2010).

Theory summary: Schemas

Different types of schema have been identified (Fiske and Taylor, 1991).

- *Self-schemas* have to do with knowledge of ourselves.
- *Event schemas* (or *scripts*) relate to the sequence of events characterising particular, frequently encountered, situations, such as buying an item from a shop, organising a doctor's appointment or arranging a holiday.
- *Role schemas* guide our expectations of how people should behave according to unspoken rules of gender, race, class, power and influence.
- *Causal schemas* enable us to form judgements about the relationship between cause and effect in our material and social environment, and to adopt problem-solving strategies based on these judgements.
- *Person schemas* enable us to make a judgement about the social categories to fit other people into.

It is useful to think of schemas lying dormant, in the sense that we are not always consciously aware of their influence on our emotions, thinking and behaviour. However, there are times when our personal schemas can be activated so that we are more 'in touch' with them (for example, the negatively held self-schema 'I am useless' or 'I am worthless' may be activated at times of acute stress). Equally, our personally held schemas may be violated (for example, getting into trouble over something when you believe that you've done nothing wrong and that you are a fundamentally good person). Finally, the actions of others may activate the schemas we hold about either other people generally or particular groups of people.

Activity 2.5   *Decision making*

Imagine that, for the first time in your life, you have been stopped by a policeman who accuses you of speeding while driving. With the different types of schemas in mind, from the theory summary box above, consider what schemas about yourself and/or others have been either activated or violated, or both.

Hint: This activity is aimed to help you see the factors at play in schema activation and/or violation. The perspective that we are all at the mercy of our schemas may help you reconsider your previously held beliefs that human beings were either 'good' or 'bad'.

In relation to the notion that we should embrace non-judgementalism, it should be clear by now that the human ability to make short-cut judgements has clear advantages and disadvantages. From Activity 2.5, on the one hand, it may be apparent that it is to our advantage to expect what kind of interpersonal encounter is likely to happen in situations where there are clear contextual, situational and relational cues to determine behaviour (Hargie and Dickson, 2004).

On the other hand, it is equally likely that many of us will make judgements based on prejudice-related stereotyping (Oakes et al., 1994; Tourish, in Long, 1999; Hargie and Dickson, 2004; Augoustinos et al., 2014). When we stereotype others, we place them in general categories and ignore their individual characteristics. The cost of this is that *we fail to appreciate the complete uniqueness of the whole person, ensuring that our stereotypes sometimes lead us into judgements that are both erroneous and biased* (Tourish, in Long, 1999, p193).

To be discussed and developed more in Chapter 6, it is a fact that stereotypes are widely held about social groups and individual people. It is also clear that stereotypes can become self-fulfilling. For example, if a nurse regards all shaven-headed men as aggressive, she or he might act towards them in a defensively belligerent way. This may well precipitate an aggressive reaction from them which, in a circular way, will confirm the nurse's stereotype.

Activity 2.6   *Reflection*

Take a few minutes to consider whether there are any individuals, or groups of individuals, whom you have a prejudice towards. Having identified an individual or a group, consider what sources of information you are using to inform your prejudice. Equally, think about the things that you don't know about the individual or group that may have a bearing on you sustaining or dropping your prejudice about them.

Hint: All of us develop prejudices as a result of the ways in which we were socialised to life and other people in our early years. Some of us maintain our prejudices by limiting the kinds and sources of information about the world that we expose ourselves to – for example, by only reading a particular newspaper.

Case study: Challenging behaviour as communication

Gillian, a first-year student nurse, is sitting in a day room, beside a young woman with learning difficulties. The woman grabs at Gillian's wrist. Gillian feels upset and starts to experience stereotypical thoughts corresponding to a widely held view that clients with learning difficulties are aggressive. The service user continues to pull at Gillian's wrist and starts making screeching noises. After a little while, Gillian allows herself to be led by the client, who takes her into the kitchen and towards the tap. Gillian realises that she simply wanted a drink, and later takes the trouble to find out more about the function of challenging behaviour as a form of communication.

Prejudice and related stereotyping are particularly relevant problems for interpersonal communication in nursing. As described above, if a nurse, for example, acts towards a patient 'as if' he or she were completely like the stereotype the nurse imagines, the patient is likely to respond in possibly a defensive or angry way, often because the patient is aware that he or she has been unjustly 'put in a box'. The patient's behaviour may then confirm to the nurse that the nurse's (prejudiced, stereotyping) attitude was correct and the nurse may not be sufficiently aware of the fact that he or she is acting towards the patient on the basis of unfair and inappropriate judgemental attitudes.

Given the inevitability of making instant contextual evaluations about people, and their advantages and disadvantages, it seems more reasonable for people to strive towards becoming more constantly and critically aware of the judgements they are making about people rather than trying to be 'non-judgemental' in Burnard's (1996) sense. Critical awareness of such judgements can also, helpfully, contribute to their modification when nurses try to get to know the person behind the stereotype. This requires nurses to practise in a **metacognitive** manner (Hargie and Dickson, 2004) – in other words, to think about the ways in which they think about other people.

Self-awareness and empathy

A further question for nurses considering the viability of the humanistic approach for CIPS is: how useful is the concept of **self-awareness** for their practice? It is often argued (for example, see McCabe and Timmins, 2006, 2013) that self-awareness is a significant tool for improving nurse–patient interaction and should be an integral part of nurse education. In this vein, based on the inherent benefits of being self-aware, it is equally asserted that self-awareness is essential for the successful implementation of the therapeutic relationship (McCabe and Timmins, 2006, 2013). Others have flagged up the importance of its use in the professional and personal development of nurses (see, for example, Burnard, 1996; McCabe and Timmins, 2006, 2013). In a style very characteristic of the durability of an uncritical acceptance of the 'self-awareness' principle in the nursing CIPS literature over the years, Kagan et al. (1986, p21) stated that:

> *self-awareness is central to interpersonal skill. We use knowledge about ourselves to plan our part in any interaction, and to put these plans into practice: our past experience contributes to our attitudes and values and affects what we notice about other people's behaviour and how we interpret it. Understanding our reactions to what others say and do will help us to relate more effectively to them.*

In the light of the above, and the discussion that preceded it, it may not be unreasonable to assume that it is important to strive towards being as aware as possible of our attitudes, beliefs about others and behaviour towards them. However, a fundamental problem with the self-awareness concept is with regard to assumptions of the nature of 'the self' (Holstein and Gubrium, 2000). The notion of the coherent, single and developing self belongs to the philosophical tradition that gave rise to humanistic psychology in the mid-twentieth century, and to related counselling and psychotherapeutic principles and interventions.

However, in line with theoretical and empirical work in contemporary social psychology (Holstein and Gubrium, 2000; Augoustinos et al., 2014) and human and social science (Grant, 2010c, 2013), it is arguably more useful for us to consider ourselves to be often contradictory, multiple selves, rather than coherent and predictable single selves. From this perspective, each one of us is likely to act in different, sometimes surprising and contradictory ways (to both ourselves and others), in different social contexts, thus behaving and experiencing ourselves and others inconsistently over time.

The importance of sensitivity to often complex social contexts, and to the corresponding shifting experiences of self and others, has interrelated implications for nurses who wish to practise safe and effective CIPS that adhere in a balanced way to evidence-based principles. First, nurses should try to be constantly mindful of contextual factors within which relationships with patients/clients are embedded (Hargie and Dickson, 2004), rather than inflexibly trying to adhere to a prescriptive set of communication rules and expectations of context-free and predictable selves, which, by default, will ignore contextual factors.

Second, given the discussion above, nurses need to be mindful of the lack of context in narrow or conventional readings of **evidence-based practice** generally, including that which informs CIPS specifically (Hargie and Dickson, 2004; Brown et al., 2006). McCabe and Timmins argued that:

> *[the use of the] principles of good communication . . . rather than nurses in the health care setting using static models of communication, results in more effective patient-centred communication . . . Several contemporary authors contend that current theories of nursing and models of nursing are inadequate to inform the complexity of healthcare situations.*
> (McCabe and Timmins, 2006, p167)

Essentially, McCabe and Timmins argue against a 'one model fits all' approach to both evidence-based practice and related forms of communication and interpersonal relating. Rather, nurses should always be mindful of, and respond to, the individual meaning and context of each interpersonal situation in complex shifting healthcare environments.

The organisational climate

Based on a review of the literature, and theoretical and empirical work, Reynolds and Scott (2000) contextually locate empathy in the interpersonal climate of the healthcare setting. Patients need to feel safe in their relationships and this depends on the development of trust. In these authors' judgement, trust in this context depends on the promotion of a culture of warmth and genuineness (or honesty) on the part of the nurse, in order for disclosure and non-judgemental exploration of the patient's experiences and feelings to occur. This highlights the importance of the evidence-based need to look at the organisational conditions influencing and determining the form and content of interpersonal communication in nursing.

From this basis, it might be reasonable to pose the question: what happens when the interpersonal context and climate work against the development and practice of empathy? Supporting the contemporary work on social cognition discussed earlier, in particular the exercise of the five types of schema (self, event, role, causal and person) and stereotyping, Rogers (1961) argued that a barrier to exploration of feelings is a very natural tendency to evaluate, disapprove and judge. This seems especially to be the case when a patient's communication is ambiguous or threatening. In these circumstances, nurses can become:

defensive, often transmitting this to the client through unwanted advice, failure to respond to direct questions, or curt unfriendly voice tone . . . [according to Rogers] . . . the logical means of correcting this tendency is to work on achieving genuineness . . . once this is established, the work of helping proceeds through the helper's moment-by-moment empathic grasp of the meaning and significance of the client's world.
(Reynolds and Scott, 2000, p229)

Research summary: Teaching empathy

Work on achieving genuineness in order to enhance a nurse's ability to be empathic begs the question of how empathy is taught. Howe (2013) provides a good discussion of examples of good practice in teaching empathy across a range of populations and disciplines, including healthcare and helping professionals. However, based on a review of the literature, Reynolds and Scott (2000) argued that empathy training in nurse education is limited by a failure to define empathy specifically and to locate it within an interpersonal theory. They also assert that a further problem for empathy education is related to its value for the realities of clinical practice, and conclude that there is a need for new ways of helping nurses to develop their abilities to express empathy in clinical contexts because of the low levels of empathy in nursing and the limitations of existing empathy courses. Among other conclusions from the literature reviewed, they highlighted that:

- the optimum length of an empathy course is unclear;
- there is no common agreement about which components of an empathy course are effective;
- it is unclear what the long-term consequences of empathy training are for nurse–patient relationships;
- empathy education needs to have relevance to the clinical circumstances in which it really matters;
- therefore, clinically focused education may provide nurses with a more meaningful development of empathy skills.

First- and second-level forms of communication

Morse et al. (1992) discussed the differences between nurses behaving in a client/patient-focused or **nurse-focused** way and whether the communication was spontaneous (which Morse et al. called *first-level*) or learned (termed *second-level*). According to these authors, client/patient-focused, first-level communication is emotionally driven and culturally conditioned and, therefore, is often an unconscious response on the part of the nurse. This type of communication includes responses such as pity, sympathy, consolation, compassion, commiseration and reflexive reassurance. This is often regarded as normal, everyday communication, but is often undervalued and seen as superficial.

Patient-focused, second-level (learned) communication includes responses such as sharing self, confronting, humour and informative reassurance. This is an important form of communication, but it is vital that the interaction is, relatively speaking, focused on the client/patient rather than the nurse (although nurses do have to give some information about themselves).

Nurse-focused, first-level responses include guarding, dehumanising, withdrawing, distancing, labelling and denying, often rationalised within the 'busy nurse' persona (see Chapter 1). Deriving in large part from the work of Menzies Lyth (1988), these can be conscious or unconscious responses that nurses use to detach from difficult or emotionally demanding situations in order to cope with stress or very intense feelings. This results in task- rather than patient-focused work, which tends to isolate patients/clients, making them feel more anxious and lonely. Along with task-focused work comes a reduction in good CIPS.

Nurse-focused, second-level communication includes rote or mechanical responses, false pity and false reassurance. Nurses who communicate in this way can appear distant and uncaring to their patients, making the patients feel undervalued. This, in turn, lowers the self-esteem of patients (Fennell, 1999) and may undermine the trust that they have for nurses and their willingness to talk with nurses about how they are feeling, either physically or psychologically. Second-level communication is characterised by conversation closure statements on the part of the nurses, such as 'don't worry' and 'everything will be fine'. Patients may thus begin to believe that they are over-reacting to their own illnesses. Nurses may, consciously or unconsciously, use this form of communication to prevent patients from verbalising any further fears (Menzies Lyth, 1988). At a conscious level, this may be done because nurses genuinely feel that they don't have the time to listen. However, at an unconscious level, conversation closure behaviour on the part of nurses may mean that the emotions behind their patients' questions are too intense to deal with.

Case study: 'Fobbing off' a patient

Jack is a first-year student in the mental health field, on a practice learning experience in an acute admission ward. He is approached by Jim, a client in his late 50s, who is concerned about distressing possible side-effects of the new medication he is taking. Jim, clearly scared about what's happening to him physically, has asked Jack several times that morning if his symptoms could be the side-effects of the medication. Jack is aware that the qualified staff are busy on other things, which makes him think that Jim is making an unnecessary fuss over nothing. Because of this, Jack's stock response to Jim is 'Don't worry; everything's going to be fine.' Jim is left frustrated and even more scared. This increases his reassurance-seeking behaviour with Jack, which, in turn, increases Jack's belief that Jim really is a nuisance.

Organisational environmental threats to interpersonal nursing interventions

From an environmental perspective, you can see from the discussion so far that the settings that nurses work in often do not lend themselves to the time, consistency and effort required to support patients with CIPS based on counselling or psychotherapeutic interventions. This is because of the following interrelated reasons. First, it has long been recognised in the literature of organisational theory that, in spite of realist (see Chapter 1) claims to the contrary by particular organisations, their members may be socialised into tacitly held rules of the organisation that favour custom, practice and tradition, and are thus antagonistic to the uptake and development of either narrow- or broad-reading evidence-based approaches (Pfeffer, 1981; Smircich, 1983; Richardson, 1997; Grant, 2000; Morgan, 2006; Grant and Leigh-Phippard, 2014).

Second, the kind of counselling intervention approaches favoured by advocates of Rogerian principles have often been criticised on the grounds of 'naive humanism'. This means that simply trying to create the facilities of empathy, unconditional positive regard and congruence between staff members, and between staff and patients, is unlikely to lead to the level of effective and good CIPS desired by staff. This is because real or perceived organisational imperatives, such as busyness, lack of time or technical tasks, are likely to get in the way (Brown et al., 2006), and because the implicit, conscious and unconsciously held rules of the organisation governing interpersonal, including staff–patient, relationships frequently trump practice based on humanistic principles (Menzies Lyth, 1988; Grant et al., 2011; Grant and Leigh-Phippard, 2014).

Because of such organisational rules, custom, practice and imperatives, and because of broader trends in contemporary society favouring brief communication, Brown and his colleagues argue that counselling and psychotherapy-based communication and interpersonal models have become increasingly old-fashioned.

Blip culture communication

Drawing on the work of Toffler (1980), Brown et al. (2006) argue that we live in a time they describe as characterised by **blip culture** forms of interpersonally relating. This means that the leisurely conversations of the past (if such a time ever existed for nurses) were possible only because the organisational context of nursing practice allowed for this. In their view, blip culture health organisational members now only have time for brief interpersonal exchanges with their patients. Although this situation is lamentable, the challenge for nurses is to make these brief exchanges effective and empathic in the light of the preceding discussion.

Implications for nursing practice

In conclusion, the following interrelated set of evidence-based principles for the increasingly skilled practice of interpersonal communication has emerged from the preceding discussion.

Nurses would do well to consider the limitations of a sole investment in humanistic, counselling models of CIPS. A more empirically sound approach, based on a considered amalgam of narrow and broad readings of EBP, suggests that the person–situation context of communication is crucial.

Metacognitive practice by nurses (or thinking about how they think about the ways in which they communicate and interpersonally relate to their patients) will enable exploration of the way they think about patient groups and how such styles of thinking came about. This may include the personal characteristics of communication, such as self, event, role, causal or person schemas; or stereotyping; or unconsciously driven defences against intimacy with patients; or first- and second-level forms of communication. Equally, it may relate to characteristics of the organisational frameworks within which communication takes place.

Turn back to the case study of John (avoiding anger) in Chapter 1. If John is not helped to recognise and change his behaviour, how will it impact on patients, other staff and learners if he rises to the position of charge nurse? Metacognitive practice by nurses is also necessary because of the way they have been socialised into particular organisational communication styles, which may either enhance or threaten skilled interpersonal practice.

Given the principle that all communication is governed by context, and although some environments may lend themselves to – albeit unlikely – leisurely interpersonal exchanges, others are, by default, more appropriate for brief, 'blip culture' forms of communication, although great care must be taken to minimise sacrificing contextual depth in brief exchanges. Equally, some organisational contexts may promote ineffective, damaging or abusive types of communication.

From the basis of the above principles, it will be useful for nurses to practise the specifics of empathy. This includes empathy both in the interpersonal context and in the work-setting, or interpersonal climate, context. To facilitate this, clinically focused empathy education is relevant and much needed.

Chapter summary

This chapter has introduced you to key issues in the historical development of research in CIPS in nursing. It has looked at the relationship between research in CIPS and teaching and experiential learning. All communication is governed by context. There are problems in nurses having a sole reliance on humanistic counselling/psychotherapy models of communication. Schema-driven and schema-activated behaviour is relevant to the practice of good CIPS in nursing. Good interpersonal and organisational climates are relevant for the practice of good nursing CIPS.

An understanding of what is meant by patient first- and second-level forms of communication is important for nurses. You should be able to demonstrate an appreciation of the organisational environmental threats to counselling and psychotherapy nursing interventions. Finally, nurses should understand what is meant by 'blip cultures' and the opportunities and constraints for forms of communication emerging from such cultures.

Chapter 2

Activities: brief outline answers

Activity 2.1 The meaning of evidence-based healthcare in practice (p40)

Attitudes may be polarised: some colleagues will diminish or dismiss the value of lived-experience knowledge as being anecdotal, unscientific, ungrateful, sob stories, irrelevant, whereas others will describe them as central to understanding good healthcare.

Activity 2.2 Evidence-based CIPS (p41)

Writers such as Schön (1987) and Freshwater and Rolfe (2001) argue that translating research into clinical practice is far from straightforward. These authors maintained that this is because of a faulty assumption of *technical rationality* held by those (usually members of research communities) who believe that research outcomes can simply be applied in a straightforward manner in clinical settings. In critiquing this assumption, Schön (1987) uses the metaphor of the high hard ground overlooking a swamp. The high hard ground is the world where research is conducted in a relatively clean, 'sterile' way. The swampland is the messy, murky world of clinical practice where relationships and work are never straightforward and cannot be controlled to the extent that research environments are.

Further reading

Augoustinos, M, Walker, I and Donaghue, N (2014) *Social Cognition: An integrated introduction*, 3rd edn. London: Sage.

This book will provide you with contemporary evidence-based information on social cognition, and its relationship with social identity and communication.

Brown, B, Crawford, P and Carter, R (2006) *Evidence-Based Health Communication.* Maidenhead: Open University Press and McGraw-Hill Education.

This book offers a critical evaluation of the kinds of evidence that have been collected concerning both effective communication and the training health professionals receive in communication.

Charon, R (2001) Narrative medicine: a model for empathy, reflection, profession, and trust. *Journal of the American Medical Association*, 286(15): 1897–1902.

This is an important paper in arguing the case for narrative competency in healthcare professionals.

Useful website

http://psychology.wikia.com/wiki/Social_Cognition_Paper_Archive_and_Information_Centre

This is the website of the Psychology Wiki Social Cognition Paper Archive and Information Center. There are lots of downloads and links that will interest readers accessing this site.

Chapter 3
The safe and effective practice of communication and interpersonal skills

NMC Standards for Pre-registration Nursing Education

This chapter will address the following competencies:

Domain 2: Communication and interpersonal skills
1. All nurses must build partnerships and therapeutic relationships through safe, effective and non-discriminatory communication. They must take account of individual differences, capabilities and needs.
5. All nurses must use therapeutic principles to engage, maintain and, where appropriate, disengage from professional caring relationships, and must always respect professional boundaries.

NMC Essential Skills Clusters

This chapter will address the following ESCs:

Cluster: Care, compassion and communication
2. People can trust the newly registered graduate nurse to engage in person-centred care empowering people to make choices about how their needs are met when they are unable to meet them for themselves.

By the first progression point:
1. Takes a person-centred, personalised approach to care.

By the second progression point:
2. Actively empowers people to be involved in the assessment and care planning process.

Introduction

It is generally agreed that CIPS underpin effective and safe relationships. In order to understand the nature of nurse–patient relationships, it is valuable to take time to appreciate the spectrum of those that can occur within nurses' professional lives. For example, relationships can range from providing total physical and tangible care in extreme cases of physical illness, to emotional support of an entirely invisible nature or support through, for example, professional/social encounters in a community setting. The nature of these encounters is as varied as a colour palette, and different nurses in different settings, such as caring for adults or children, in mental health settings or with clients with learning disabilities, may experience more or less of one particular area of the palette. But, in all likelihood, there will be elements of this palette in all your interpersonal relationships with patients.

Knowing how to respond and react in these many situations can be bewildering if you have to imagine how you will manage these different forms of relationships in order to be effective. This chapter aims to provide a guide in these situations to give you confidence as well as create a sense of self-awareness. This is a crucial ingredient of a safe and effective nurse–patient relationship. We will explore what it means to be safe and begin by examining some of the theory behind the way we think in social situations and how that influences how we behave. Called the **social thinking** processes, these are the hidden thought processes by which people process and interpret information from and about themselves (their intrapersonal world) and other persons (their interpersonal world).

The roles we take on in relationships and the phases of the nurse–patient relationship play a large part in achieving a clear and effective communication process. This chapter will explore the many roles you have within and beyond the professional settings. The fundamental core general skills that are needed in CIPS will be explained and demonstrated in practical, work-based contexts. The chapter concludes by discussing the phases of the nurse–patient relationship and by comparing two models. There is a discussion of the nature of the helping relationship in nursing and the notion that this relationship can have a therapeutic effect. The patient's role in decision making in the nurse–patient relationship is analysed in respect of recent health policy.

What does 'being safe' mean?

'Being safe' is a term used to describe how nurse–patient relationships can be conducted without either party being harmed. Our professional duty is to ensure that service users are safe. This is enshrined in standard 1, section 3 of the NMC *Standards for Pre-registration Nursing Education*, the purpose of which is:

> *To establish the essential safeguards on any action or act of omission committed or witnessed by a nursing or midwifery student that affects the safety or wellbeing of service users.*
> (NMC, 2010, p49)

From the start of your training, you have a duty to provide care safely at all times and people must be able to trust you with their lives and their health. To justify that, the *Standards* are clear that you must *act to safeguard the public, and be responsible and accountable for safe, person-centred, evidence-based nursing practice* (p5). In order to progress through the course, a criterion for the first progression point in the *Standards* covers *safety, safeguarding and protection of people of all ages, their carers and their families* (p97). Specifically, you must demonstrate *safe, basic, person-centred care, under supervision, for people who are unable to meet their own physical and emotional needs* within the domain of communication and interpersonal skills (p98).

With this in mind, we have to be careful not to cause harm, injury or damage in our communication and interpersonal relationships with patients. How can we do that with words, you may be asking? Well, as we know, words are powerful objects that shape the messages we are sending. How we interpret the messages is where the damage may start.

The interpretation of the meanings of words varies from person to person. In addition, we are dealing in healthcare with many words that are unfamiliar to patients until they have understood and learned their meaning. This applies to the names of conditions as well as the phrases and abbreviations we use as short cuts to describe objects, processes, procedures and situations.

The way in which we transmit the words in our messages can be influenced by many factors, as discussed in previous chapters. Information transmission has to be interpreted and assimilated by both parties in the interaction. Our body language and non-verbal signals can all lead to misunderstanding and confusion if they are not correctly understood by the patient. This is further complicated by the anxiety patients may have about their health, their previous experiences of healthcare and the relative success of those experiences, their cultural or personalised view of the world and the degree of discomfort or pain they may be experiencing during the communication. These are the distracting stimuli described by Bateson (1979) in the circular model of communication, introduced in Chapter 1.

It is not only the interpretation the patient may place on the messages that is important. You, as a nurse, need to interpret patients' responses correctly, so that you know how much they understand about the situation and are sure that they have understood what you are saying or are intending to do. Your interpretation is therefore equally relevant.

Scenario 1

The pattern goes like this:

1. *The student nurse tells the patient that he must have a shower at 6 in preparation for a surgical procedure. The patient is to undergo a routine procedure and has no major health problems.*
2. *The patient nods, indicating he has understood. The patient has interpreted this as taking a shower at 6 p.m., whereas the student nurse meant 6 a.m. So this is a semi-correct interpretation of the message. The patient is conscious of his health and keeps himself fit and well; however, he is frightened of falling in the shower and does not have a shower at home. At home he has a seat in the bath and uses a shower attachment. The student nurse looks very busy and the patient does not want to be a nuisance, so he does not ask for clarification. The patient is worried about the surgery and has not slept well, so his receptivity of information is compromised by tiredness and anxiety.*
3. *Because the patient nodded in apparent agreement, the student nurse says something like 'That's OK then' and goes to the next patient.*

It's not difficult to anticipate what will happen next. The patient will not have the shower at the correct time. If the student nurse does spot this in time, the patient will take a long time because he is nervous of falling in the shower; he may even fall because he is unaccustomed to using a shower. The surgery is delayed; the operating theatre's schedule is put back, causing inconvenience to patients and staff alike. If the patient were to fall, the surgery would probably be cancelled and the patient would suffer more, in addition to enduring the delayed solution to his original problem.

Let's try it again.

Scenario 2

The pattern goes like this:

1. *The student nurse tells the patient that he has to prepare for surgery (this tells the patient what the communication is all about) that morning (this tells the patient when it is going to happen). The patient needs to have a shower at 6 a.m. (It might seem obvious to state the time as this communication is taking place in the morning, but it makes it clearer and reinforces the time frame for the patient.)*
2. *The student nurse asks the patient if he is comfortable having a shower or is there any other way that he usually has a full wash? (This gives the patient the opportunity to express his personal hygiene methods and confirm that he can shower or describe what he needs to do.)*
3. *The patient responds by explaining how he usually washes.*

4. *The student nurse needs to find out not only how, but why, the patient washes in this manner. This can shed light on any fear of falling.*

5. *The student nurse explores how the facilities on the ward can be adapted to suit the patient and checks whether the patient agrees. As the environment is unfamiliar to the patient and his usual routine is disrupted, it would be additionally helpful if the student nurse were to take the patient to the shower facilities and demonstrate to him how to use the shower.*

6. *During this encounter, the student nurse can explore with the patient any concerns or anxieties he may have about the preparations for surgery, such as falling in the shower, and at the same time clarify any fears about the surgical procedure, if these have not already been elicited during the assessment processes. This takes additional time, but could avoid a great deal of future inconvenience and potential safety issues. It could also provide opportunities to develop the nurse's relationship with the patient and understand his current needs, as well as prepare for their communication postoperatively.*

These scenarios illustrate how a simple communication request can involve several aspects of meeting physical and emotional needs. The success of managing these aspects is often due to our abilities to perceive and interpret information. This has been studied in a branch of social psychology termed 'social cognition', often referred to as 'social thinking'. The aim of these studies is to find out how people take in information and assimilate it so that it can be used effectively in social situations with friends and family, but the studies can also be used to improve professional relationships.

The process of social thinking

Social thinking is the process by which people assimilate and interpret information or thoughts from and about themselves (their intrapersonal world) and other individuals (their interpersonal world). Most of the time our social thinking activities work very well for us in social situations. We pay attention to the most, rather than the least, important aspects of our environment, which keeps us safe. We think about people in a way that organises our ideas into categories, so that we can recognise characteristics about people. Humans use a process of social comparison to do this. Comparing what we are encountering with what we have encountered before gives us a frame of reference or benchmark to make judgements. We can also take in all manner of facts, which originate from different sources and experiences, and organise them into categories so that we can recognise them again. Generally, we remember what we need to remember, and make conclusions about facts and ideas, all of which influences how we react and respond in situations.

Finding out more about how social thinking operates is one way to ensure we accurately understand and interpret what people around us are expressing. There is a 'recipe' for social thinking that has been built up around two of the most common types of reaction to people and events.

These are spontaneous and deliberative. Spontaneous means 'off the top of your head' responses, such as 'all experts must be right' or 'all exotic food must taste disgusting'. These quick responses mean that we have not taken the time to gather further information or evidence to verify the judgement.

At other times, people will engage in a more deliberative response, taking time to elaborate on the statement or follow different ideas that reach away from the original thought to engage with new ideas. This comes with an analysis of problems or wider impressions of a situation or context. It is where old habitual patterns of response or assumptions are reconsidered and delved into more deeply to arrive at a fuller picture of events, ideas and impressions. Based on the work of Wyer and Srull (1986), a recipe for social thinking has been designed that describes these two stages of a process that assembles impressions, conclusions, decisions and intentions.

Stage 1: Spontaneous

- *Take* raw sensations such as sights, sounds, words and sentences.
- *Add* these together to form an initial comprehension.
- *Organise* without being aware of the decisions into handy, familiar categories.
- *Integrate* with whatever you happen to be thinking of at the time.
- *Generate* new thoughts, which are organised and integrated with the original information.

These actions are undertaken as quickly and as automatically as possible and could be the final impression, conclusion, decision or intention. Often, this is as far as people get in the recipe, because it is a quick and easy method.

If, on the one hand, the topic is not important, or they have other more pressing things to do, or they are not particularly close to the person or persons involved in the situation, the process stops here. If, on the other hand, they are more interested, are closely involved in the outcome of the situation or committed in some way – that is, more willing and able to do so – they will progress to the second stage of the process.

Stage 2: Deliberative

- *Use* your current goals or aims, or what you want to achieve in the situation.
- *Apply* your general world-view knowledge, schemas from your personal previous experiences or underpinning research evidence.
- *Apply* your knowledge of people's expectations of what they want to achieve and how they would go about it in this situation.
- *Apply* your knowledge of the specific individuals, groups, communities and other situations such as this one that you may not have experienced personally.

There is no order in applying these deliberations; they are merely different types of knowledge that you can draw upon to assimilate information about a patient. The finished product of these deliberations is a final summary of impressions, conclusions, decisions or intentions. This may confirm an initial impression; however, it may be adjusted or altered from the initial view. The process of deeper analysis does not have to take a long time, but gathering together additional information upon which to make a judgement can provide a safer and more informed way to proceed in a nurse–patient relationship that is not based solely upon initial judgements.

Cognitive stores

Students are often surprised that experienced staff can draw conclusions about complex situations or seem to have an intuitive understanding of patients' needs, without the patients appearing to have directly expressed those needs. One explanation for this is that experienced staff have a store of previous experiences, knowledge of different societal groups and up-to-date knowledge of contemporary research that they synthesise rapidly to form their conclusions. Their spontaneous recipe works for them. However, even the most experienced staff have occasions when they have to reflect on their judgements to ensure that they are not using habitual stereotypes or outdated research to make their decisions. These are referred to as cognitive stores of information.

Cognitive misers

If staff do not use their cognitive stores effectively, they run the risk of becoming 'cognitive misers'. Cognitive misers do not put effort into thinking around the problem or situation, and only use the minimum cognitive resources they need. A consequence of this is that some knowledge becomes so automatic that it is incorporated into the organising part of the recipe without any extra effort ever being put into the deliberative stage. Vital information could be overlooked.

Recency

Another danger is the recency with which a category has been used. The more recently a category is used, the more likely it is that it will be used again. The consequence of this is that new information could be consigned to the same category, when there may be differences that are relevant to consider. This can also apply to the three types of knowledge in the deliberative stage. Combining the recency factor with the cognitive miser factor means that people will not consider other options and will stop with a 'good enough' fit.

Self-generating thoughts

One final principle to discuss is how we self-generate our thoughts in the final part of the spontaneous recipe stage and the pitfalls this may provide. Even when we are tired, we generate thoughts. Our brains continue to run along by themselves even when we are in a darkened room and have little information to receive, such as the raw sensations of light, touch, heat or cold. These are self-generated thoughts that flit from one topic to another, but are organised insofar as they are recognisable to us as we compare them to the knowledge categories we have established. These thoughts are not entirely random, as they are linked to significant topics that have been thought about recently (the recency factor again) and thus can be biased towards these topics. These thoughts can also become organised and integrated into familiar categories.

We can also generate scenarios that are figments of our imagination, and our difficulty is that we cannot always distinguish between these and the information that is drawn from the raw sensations in the first stage of the recipe. For example, we cannot always remember whether we put the keys in their usual place or whether we imagined we did! In the same way, we cannot always differentiate between self-generated imaginings and information from actual situations. This is because the processing of the information is rapid, familiar and unconscious.

To guard against this human foible in healthcare, we need to use both spontaneous and deliberative stages in appropriate situations. When a snap judgement is required and time is not available, we make spontaneous decisions. However, to be safe and to understand and interpret our patients' needs fully, we need to communicate with them to gather information in the spontaneous stage that we can then feed into the deliberative stage. The summary from the first stage is combined with different types of knowledge in the second stage to make an informed assessment of the patients' understanding of how their health needs can be met.

Case study: From spontaneous to deliberative social thinking

Rani is a first-year children's nurse at the start of her morning shift. She passes the bed of Jamie, a five-year-old boy with asthma-related problems. She cheerily waves and says 'Hiya Jamie, I see your football team won this weekend', and is about to move on when she notices that Jamie looks more serious than usual. She then, momentarily, becomes aware that the kind of greeting that she has given Jamie is part of a start-of-shift ritual that she and other members of staff engage in with all the children in their care, without stopping to focus attention on any one child in particular. Because of this, instead of going on to greet the other children, she sits by Jamie's bed. 'What's up, Jamie? You don't look your usual perky self', she asks. Jamie then discloses that he wants to be a professional footballer when he grows up, but worries that he never will because of his problems. Rani mentally consults her knowledge and research base about recovery from childhood respiratory problems before proceeding to reassure him sensitively but positively.

Most nurse–patient interactions share features with social interactions generally, in being dynamic, creative, responsive and socially constructed. The primary mode of communication is talk enhanced with gestures, personal communication style and body language. This enables the two partners to exchange information, agree decisions, and develop and maintain the relationship. However, most healthcare encounters can be thought of as an interaction between two distinct cultures (Edelman, 2000) – the medical culture and the culture of the patient.

The differences between the two cultural groups are that they think differently about health and illness, and that they have different perceptions, attitudes, types of knowledge, sources of knowledge and agendas. The patients' agendas will be based upon their expectations and experiences of illness, health, consultation and treatments, whereas the agendas of healthcare professionals are likely to reflect their own (usually western) medical or health-related training together with personal background factors. Reconciling these differences is one of the major challenges to engaging in a successful nurse–patient relationship.

One way to clarify and negotiate through this conjunction of cultures is to identify in nurse–patient interactions two basic goals: the first goal is associated with information giving and responding to questions, and the second with relationship building. Separating out these goals within interactions can help clarify what will be gained from the interaction. Information giving and responding to question activities are related to adherence, or following instructions, and remembering information, whereas patient satisfaction is related to the socio-emotional aspects of interactions. Despite our best efforts at good communication, patients report the highest levels of dissatisfaction over poor communication in clinical settings (McCabe, 2004). The areas of dissatisfaction found in McCabe's study were a lack of:

- information and a concentration on tasks rather than communicating;
- readiness to listen or attend demonstrated with body language;
- empathetic responses that alleviated anxiety and uncertainty through emotional engagement;
- friendliness and some humour that helps to relax, creating a social function that helps to pass the time.

For the nurse, there may be a desire for the patient to achieve a satisfactory understanding of procedures and processes, whereas the patient may wish to have satisfaction from receiving kindness, empathy and a sense of respect. Alternatively, patients may want information and nurses may want recognition for the work they are doing. Achieving a balance in reaching these respective goals is needed. The responsibility for understanding the balance lies with the nurse, which is why differentiating between the **professional relationship** and the **social relationship** is necessary. This is discussed further in the following chapter.

Case study: Achieving a balance between the two basic goals

Django is a first-year student nurse on a practice learning experience with two community staff nurses, Erica and Chen-Chi. He notices that Erica seems keen to see as many patients as she can in the shortest possible time. Her typical style is to arrive at a patient's home, observe the minimal demands of courtesy before eliciting information from the patient about the problem, provide the appropriate nursing intervention, with instructions, if appropriate, then leave. In contrast, Chen-Chi takes her time and seems to privilege developing empathic and supportive relationships with her patients as an essential part of good community nursing care. Django notices that Chen-Chi's patients reciprocate warmth to her. This contrasts with Erica's patients, who look uncomfortable in her presence.

Roles

We all have several roles: some examples are daughter, brother, friend, companion, partner, parent, colleague, manager and subordinate. How many roles do you have? They all require different identities and yet they are often linked. There are occasions when roles can overlap and, in some cases, form parts of, or belong to, a particular social identity. In general, you will have a small number of primary roles and a significantly larger number of secondary roles. Maintaining a social identity as a nurse requires acceptance of the role and an ability to relate to other nurses. Yet within nursing there are other specialties that involve different types of relationship. For example, critical care nurses relate in a different way to their patients when compared with mental health nurses and their clients. The context and requirements of the roles are different. But that is not to say that critical care nurses do not relate to emotional issues (for example, see Peel, 2003, on breaking bad news to relatives on critical care units) or dealing with emergency mental health conditions (for example, see Broadbent et al., 2002, who devised a triage assessment tool specifically to deal with mental health emergencies in a unit where 2.6 per cent of all admissions had primary mental health issues).

Activity 3.1   *Reflection*

Draw a network diagram of your roles (see example below).

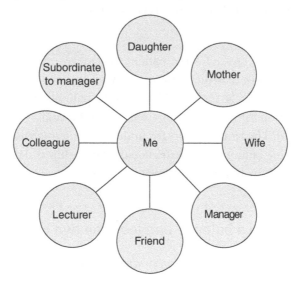

- Which are primary and secondary roles?
- Which role do you think defines you the most?

The literature suggests that social roles (i.e. roles that require taking on role-appropriate behaviours defined by rules and relationships) are where we take on a social identity but where this identity may not be our defining identity.

There are times when you may feel a conflict between roles that you have – such as being a student, which is a childlike role, and yet being beyond childhood, which is an adult role. Understanding this concept and maintaining a sense of self-identity when we are in challenging professional roles (for example, are you feeling like a nurse or a parent in a situation?) can help to manage role confusion and blurring of roles. So your answer to which role defines you most should be that your primary role may be influenced by one of your secondary roles, but the real you will be a unique and separate set of characteristics.

Now draw a diagram of a practice learning experience you undertook recently and include all the roles you observed there. Identify what characteristics, rules and expectations define those roles – not forgetting the patient in this analysis.

- How much does clothing define the role? Or hierarchies of responsibilities?
- Are there traditions, rituals, myths and legends associated with the roles?
- Where are role boundaries traversed? Is this safe practice?

Discuss your thoughts and answers on these questions with your fellow students.

Phases of the nurse–patient relationship

While there are no specific rules to guide the formation or stages of relationships, we can see from our previous discussions that various cultures, societies and groups have norms that guide how relationships and roles within those relationships should be conducted. In a healthcare setting, a slightly different set of rules applies and the roles are therefore going to differ from those appropriate for a social setting. The main reason for this is that the purpose is not social, but professional. The rate at which the relationship is formed will also be different and determined by different settings. In a pre-assessment surgical assessment unit you may have only half an hour, whereas on a medical ward a patient may stay for a number of days. Children may have short or long periods of time in hospital. In mental health settings there will be longer time frames within which to build indepth relationships, and in community settings the context of being in the patients' own homes provides a different pace for the stages of relationships to develop. In residential settings with learning disability clients, relationships have an even longer time span in which to develop. In relation to all of these possibilities, we will now look at two examples of specific relationship models.

Six-stage model of relationship formation

A six-stage model of relationship formation was proposed by DeVito (2007). Having such a model in mind enables the nurse to see how the relationship will develop and will give structure to the interaction, whether over a long or short period of time. Having a structure gives both nurse and patient greater clarity, and can reduce confusion over how long a relationship should last and what might be expected at each stage of the relationship. The six stages are: *contact, involvement, intimacy* and *deterioration,* which can then lead to either *repair* or *dissolution.*

In the first stage, there is perceptual *contact* during which first impressions are made. Physical appearance, friendliness, warmth and openness are noted. This quickly leads into interactional contact during which opening words are offered in the form of a welcome or greeting and involve ordinary conversation. Burnard (2003) has called these openings *phatic* conversations, within which ordinary social exchanges and small talk help to ease situations and develop rapport with patients. The nurse's demeanour and style set the tone for this and future conversations.

Involvement is where a sense of connection and mutuality are established. Questions and answers are exchanged to establish likes and similarities or the reasons for being in a situation.

Intimacy, in social settings, is where friendships, companionship and loving relationships are formed. In a professional relationship this is where closeness and levels of appropriate touch and deeper emotional connectedness through empathy and understanding are experienced. In Watson's (1988) transpersonal theory of nursing, she suggests that nurses can become so close to patients that they experience a kind of presencing, or 'being with' patients. This can happen in circumstances when patients are dying or in the extreme stages of illness.

The *deterioration* phase of the model is when the parties disengage and the end of the relationship is ahead. In the professional sense, this is where patients or clients are preparing to be discharged from care and they may reduce conversations or not explore their healthcare questions with such frequency. This is an inevitable phase of the nurse–patient relationship. If patients tend towards over-dependency in the relationship with their nurse, steps have to be taken to alter the intimacy of the interactions so that the patient grows accustomed to the withdrawal of contact.

If patients return to the ward or unit, a process of relationship *repair* takes place and participants go back to a previous stage and work forwards again. The final stage is relationship *dissolution*, which involves patients being discharged from care or, in some cases, the death of a patient. Because of the levels of intimacy a nurse can experience through these stages, managing the closeness and remaining emotionally intact can pose challenges even to the most experienced nurse.

It is worth mentioning that these stages are not only relevant to nurse–patient relationships. Nurses are also in contact with patients' relatives, friends and carers. Often the nurse will establish a relationship with persons close to the patient that will go through similar stages, and a marginally different relationship will emerge. Such relationships, always professional, will continue to have the purpose of returning the patient to health, or maintaining or promoting health.

Case study: Ending a relationship

Arya is a first-year student nurse who is undertaking a practice learning experience in a mental health day care facility.

She has developed a close relationship with Natasha, a young client who is the same age as her. Natasha started attending the facility just after Arya began her practice experience. Natasha was scared at first, but settled in quickly, mainly because Arya took an interest in her and helped her make better sense of the distressing experiences that had led to her referral.

Arya has told Natasha that she is coming to the end of her practice experience and will soon be leaving. Natasha is sad because she regards Arya as her closest friend, and wonders what she will do without her. She is scared to tell Arya this, however, as she worries that Arya will think she is silly. Arya has picked up on Natasha's dejection and gently prompts Natasha to voice her feelings and concerns. After listening to Natasha, Arya shares with her that the feelings of fondness are mutual, and also that she believes that their relationship has enabled Natasha to develop confidence in herself that will serve her well in developing future relationships with others. Together, they explore what specific things Natasha might do to achieve this and they also plan to have lunch together to celebrate both their relationship and the significance of its ending.

Theory summary: Transpersonal theory of caring

Watson's theory of transpersonal caring (Watson, 1988; Watson and Foster, 2003) is useful to consider in this context. It is organised around concepts such as transpersonalism, phenomenology, the self and the caring occasion, with ten curative factors that guide nursing care. The theory is intended to encompass the whole of nursing; however, it places most emphasis on the experiential, interpersonal processes between the caregiver and recipient. It focuses on caring as a therapeutic relationship and attempts to reduce the components of caring to describable parts, so that these parts can be understood and learned. As such, the theory could be criticised for being reductionist. However, reduction of theory to its component parts also enables a complex phenomenon to be understood, and this is where tension exists between reductionism and explanation. The theory claims to allow for, and be open to, **existential-phenomenological** and spiritual dimensions of caring and healing that cannot be fully explained scientifically through the western mind of modern society. More information on the theory can be obtained from the web resources found at the end of the chapter.

The helping relationship

Within the relationship stages outlined above, the nurse will engage in specific techniques to assist and help the patient. This is termed the 'therapeutic relationship'. According to Henderson

(1967, px), this involves *the practice of those nursing activities which have a healing effect or those which result in movement towards health or wellness.*

McMahon's (1993) view is that nursing centres on the nurse–patient relationship and involves both overt and non-visible caring techniques:

- developing the nurse–patient relationship based upon partnership, intimacy and reciprocity;
- manipulating the environment – from the macro (organisational) level, through to the meso (patient environment) level to the micro environment (i.e. the physical features that impact on the well-being of the patient);
- teaching – involving patient education and information;
- providing comfort – physical and non-physical care;
- adopting complementary health practices – these are creative approaches to healing that are incorporated into nursing care;
- utilising tested physical interventions – incorporating intuitive approaches to care that can be supported by inductive research approaches.

To help nurses to carry out this aspect of their relationship with patients requires a deeper level of interaction that involves not only CIPS, but an integration of their knowledge of several domains, for example, physical, social and psychological. Complementing the discussion so far is Egan's (1998) skilled helper model, a framework that assists nurses to conceptualise the helping process. Egan's skilled helper model, which can be linked to Rogers' core conditions of genuineness, respect and empathy, provides a map for exploring relationships. It also creates an explicit set of techniques for managing relationships, as each will require individual adjustments to meet situations as they arise. There are three simple questions to answer in the model.

- What is going on?
- What do I want instead?
- How might I get to what I want?

Each of these questions relates to a stage in the model that can be followed sequentially but that may be used at any time. To answer any of the questions, the individual who is seeking answers tells his or her story and then explores with the helper ways to examine the options and solutions to the questions. The process involves looking at information and clarifying meanings. Early on in this chapter we talked about interpretations and perceptions and how they can exert influence. This model is a way of exploring in detail what individuals want from their healthcare and how nurses can assist them to gain the solutions they want, as well as exploring some of the realistic options to achieving better health outcomes (see useful websites at the end of the chapter for links to the model for further study).

Access the website:

www.gp-training.net/training/communication_skills/mentoring/egan.htm

Familiarise yourself with the website in relation to its aim, which is to use Egan's skilled helper model to help you in more effective problem management.

Choose either to work on your own, in relation to one of your own problems, or with a student friend in relation to his or her problem, or in relation to a problem experienced by a client or patient with whom you are working.

Work your way through the stages of the model, referring to the notes provided for each stage.

Later, consult Egan's *The Skilled Helper* book (1998) in relation to your activity notes.

Patients as decision makers

In 2006, in the context of the emergence of contemporary respect paid to the idea that patients and service users are 'experts by experience', the government launched the *Expert Patients Programme* (EPP) (Department of Health (DH), 2006). This was in response to the evidence that more people in the twenty-first century are living into their 70s, 80s and beyond. The implications are that patients will be living with long-term conditions and multiple pathologies. The programme is aimed at patients to enable them to self-manage their conditions and has a central tenet that patients understand their disease better than healthcare staff, including nurses. Patients are seen as key decision makers in their treatment processes and this is based upon experiences and research from the UK and North America. The potential of the nurse's role in assisting the EPP is to enable patients to find ways to solve difficulties and issues they have with their lifestyle and treatment regimes so that they can be in control. The self-management programme is run from local community centres. Nurses in acute and primary care settings can work in conjunction with this philosophy by adopting Egan's model, thus providing a framework to assist patients in decision making about their care. Lorig et al. (2008) evaluated the online EPP scheme and found that the programme appeared to decrease symptoms and improve health behaviours, self-efficacy and satisfaction with the healthcare system.

Activity 3.3   *Reflection*

While you are undertaking community practice experiences, you may wish to enquire about local EPPs. On the DH website (**www.dh.gov.uk**) you can use a postcode to find local programmes and you may want to contact the programme organiser and meet with him or her to find out about how the programmes are progressing and about the role of the community nurse in relation to the programmes.

Chapter summary

In this chapter we have explored the meaning of being safe and effective, without harming or being harmed, in interpersonal relationships in healthcare. We have also considered the relevance of social thinking models as explanatory frameworks and have explored the many roles in practice and the potential for role confusion. In addition, we have identified a process for communication and interrelationship skills in healthcare settings and clarified what is meant by the therapeutic relationship.

Further reading

Egan, EG (2006) *The Skilled Helper: A problem-management and opportunity development approach to helping*, 8th edn. London: Thompson Learning.

This book contains a lot of information on helping relationships, and will be a useful resource for Activity 3.2 in this chapter.

McCabe, C (2004) Nurse–patient communication: an exploration of patients' experiences. *Journal of Clinical Nursing*, 13: 41–49.

For research into patients' satisfaction with communication and the role of patient-centred care.

Useful websites

www.gp-training.net/training/communication_skills/mentoring/egan.htm
This website gives information on helping relationships.

www.watsoncaringscience.org
This is the website of the Watson Caring Science Institute and contains information on Watson's transpersonal theory.

Chapter 4
Understanding potential barriers to the safe and effective practice of communication and interpersonal skills

Introduction

This chapter explores those factors that may act as barriers and impede effective communication and interpersonal relationships. First, we investigate the shift we make in our professional work from social to professional relationships. The chapter considers how to develop safe professional relationships, by examining the different degrees of intimacy between friend and carer, and the rules of social engagement.

Next, we consider the effect that emotions can have on communication and interpersonal relationships. Emotions are a fundamental facet of human nature and our ability to express how we feel. As such, they are a vital part of our communication methods because, when we demonstrate our emotions to our friends, family and colleagues, they can recognise how we feel and tune into our emotional needs. If only it were this simple! This seemingly straightforward aspect of inter-relationships is made more complex by the need to balance our emotional expressiveness with the need to construct new ways of coping with situations and with the extent to which we express or repress our emotions. Emotions can therefore both enhance and impede communication.

Other barriers to communication that are explored in this chapter include how we construct meaning and interpret communication as a function of this construction. The effect of motivation on communicating health advice is also explored.

Finally, we consider the nature of conflict and how it arises, along with techniques to diffuse conflict in healthcare situations.

Shifting from social to professional relationships

The shift from social relationships, as we know them, to professional relationships requires a transition. This is from early social relationships based upon kinship or friendship networks to ones that are based upon professional values and governed by a code of practice. These values encompass a sense of purpose, mutuality, authenticity, empathy, active listening, confidentiality and a respect for the dignity of the patient.

This requires nurses to set aside biases, prejudices and very often their own emotions, although these very aspects of them as people arc important as they bring to the encounter the humanness that is crucial to a sound professional relationship. To help you differentiate between social and professional relationships, Table 4.1 compares some of the major elements of social and professional relationships. We will be exploring more of these elements as we go through the chapter.

Social	Professional
• You have no specific legal or professional responsibility for the person • You may be related or have a code of behaviour that is either explicitly or implicitly agreed between a group or community that provides a framework for sanctioning different codes of behaviour • Social engagement can be more informal in some instances and formal in others	• A professional has the responsibility for helping the patient regain a state of health; this involves a spectrum of activities that range from the physical to the invisible. This is governed by a professional *Code of Professional Conduct* (NMC, 2004b) • There is informality and formality in different settings and contexts • The patient and professional have to negotiate and agree the levels of formality, some of which may be dictated by the setting, e.g. a multiprofessional case review
• The purpose of the relationship is not necessarily specific or geared towards particular goals • The individuals know each other through choice, social or family connections • There is often an element of spontaneity about engaging in the relationship	• The focus of the relationship is on the needs of the patient; often engaged through necessity rather than choice • The behaviour of the professional will be planned, implemented and evaluated in a formal or semi-formal manner • The participants may not know each other • The participants may not like each other
• Feelings of liking, loving or fondness are involved and often expressed • Persons are often judgemental within the social codes of their communities or family groups about those who are beyond those groupings and may share these judgements to gain a sense of consensus in the group of group or community characteristics	• The professional seeks to be non-judgemental and non-partisan • Sharing of personal or intimate factors is unidirectional from the patient to the professional • Confidentiality is a key factor in the professional relationship

(Continued)

(Continued)

Social	Professional
• The feelings between persons in a social relationship may enhance or may detract from the relationship course	• The main aim of the professional is to guide and influence the patient towards a better understanding of the factors that are affecting the patient's health and a resolution of his or her ill-health status • The feelings of the patient are identified, acknowledged and accounted for in any discussions • The feelings of the professional are woven into the encounter to respond empathetically • It may not be appropriate to express deeper personal feelings. This is a time for careful judgement by the professional. If extreme feelings are experienced by the professional it is important to seek support from a colleague or qualified professional for guidance
• The sense of control in the relationship is more evenly shared or driven by the wants and desires of those communicating • The relationship may continue indefinitely or end depending on the degrees of mutual liking between the persons	• There is usually a planned ending to the relationship as a result of the resolution to the above factors • The professional has self- and professional knowledge through life skills and education that are deliberately brought to bear on the encounter • The professional takes responsibility for setting the boundaries of the relationship

Table 4.1: Comparison of social and professional relationships (adapted from Arnold and Boggs, 2006)

Becoming over-involved

One of the concerns professionals have is how to become involved with a patient in a sufficiently supporting manner without becoming over-involved to the extent that it is difficult to stand back and objectively assess the needs of the patient. Being ourself and bringing personal characteristics to the relationship is crucial, otherwise we would be very mechanical, rather like robots giving care. The difference is that a professional relationship, which does indeed travel a fine line between compassion on the one hand and being so close that there is an over-involvement of emotional investment on the other, has to draw a line between the two. Becoming over-involved is most likely to happen when a nurse feels an emotional connection that reminds him or her of a situation from the past, or when there are shared feelings on a matter that can have the potential to create a strong bond.

Another source of over-involvement is when a nurse feels guilty from a previous relationship in which matters were left unresolved. This could be from either a personal or a professional experience. The nurse may attempt to resolve the issues in order to make the situation feel better than the earlier one, but the danger is that the nurse may not regard the specific needs of the patient being currently cared for. Often it will be an unconscious drive that the nurse will not be aware of. This may be spotted by others who notice that the nurse is transferring her or his feelings from a previous situation to the one that is now being experienced. It takes a very self-aware person to recognise that the feelings are related to a different situation and to set them aside so that the patient's needs become uppermost. It also takes a professionally astute colleague to recognise what is happening.

Case study: Caring towards the end of life

Mary is a 79-year-old woman who has severely debilitating arthritis and is cared for in a nursing home. She is a quiet, placid woman who is widowed and has five children. Although they live some distance away, they all visit regularly, especially her two daughters and their children, who are now adults. Her favourite occupation is doing crossword puzzles.

Mary is a warm and kind person who is loved by her family. Her days are long and filled with pain from her arthritis and yet her mind is still alert and she loves to chat with the nurses. She can no longer move about on her own. She has a urinary catheter for her elimination needs, but requires regular enemas to help evacuate her bowels as the side-effects of the pain medication mean she is always constipated. She puts up with her discomforts valiantly and the nurses are noticing that she is slowly becoming sleepier each day and less interested in conversing with them. These are her twilight years.

It is very easy to become attached to this gentle, uncomplaining woman. She may be like the grandma you wish you had, or even the grandma you had and lost. If you did not have time to say goodbye to your own grandma, your relationship with Mary could be even more poignant for you. It is in this kind of situation that you have to retain your professional distance and yet still strike a balance between caring and becoming over-involved.

We looked at endings in Chapter 1, and in a situation like this endings need to be carefully and sensitively construed to avoid reliving previous emotional situations or experiencing regrets and guilt. In these kinds of circumstance, it is advisable for nurses to talk through their feelings with their mentors, clinical supervisors or colleagues to help them gain a sense of proportion.

Developing trusting relationships with colleagues with whom you can share your feelings about situations or relationships is a strategy that will ensure that you are being safe. Mentoring or supervision by senior staff are also effective methods for supporting staff who are dealing with complex situations where there are no simple solutions (Mullen, 2005).

Professional friend

The balance between being detached and over-involved is one that has to be finely struck. Bach (2004) found that community nurses developed a specific kind of professional relationship with their patients that they termed a **professional friend**. It was not a social relationship and yet it was not a detached professional relationship. This relationship was based on many of the social aspects of the relationships described above, but there did remain a fine barrier and the patients always remained on one side of that line so that the professional integrity of the nurses could remain intact. We saw in the previous chapter that in McCabe's (2004) study patients wanted nurses to be friendly. However, the invisible boundary between nurse and patient remains, even though in our current society the intimacy of personalised care and use of first names create a sense of close, social familiarity. This is never more apparent than when an issue arises in a relationship that requires the professional to act or respond in a way that would not challenge a friendship but would create an inevitable problem in a professional relationship. It is where codes of social behaviour are superseded by professional codes of, for example, confidentiality, or where harm is being done to another person that comes to light in the communications between professional and patient.

> *Professional relationships are controlled alliances that occur within a particular context and are time limited.*
> (Arnold and Boggs, 2006, p80)

In this sense, Arnold and Boggs are suggesting that the professional relationship is shaped by the professional because of the setting in which it is carried out. We would add that it is contingent on the needs of the patient. To establish and sustain interpersonal relationships, the nurse has to establish boundaries, or even constraints, that limit and ultimately make safe the interaction between patient and nurse in these settings. The boundaries are created from ethical, legal and professional codes of practice, as well as a patient's right to caring from nurses who appraise situations realistically in order to ensure responsive actions towards a patient's optimum health and well-being.

In contrast, a friendship is defined as:

> *an interpersonal relationship between two persons that is mutually productive and is characterized by mutual positive regard.*
> (DeVito, 2007, p282)

There are also thought to be three friendship types:

- *reciprocity*, characterised by loyalty, self-sacrifice, mutual affection and generosity;
- *receptivity*, characterised by a comfortable and positive imbalance in the giving and receiving of rewards; each person's needs are satisfied by the exchange;
- *association*, a transitory relationship more like a friendly relationship than a true friendship.

Your friendships, or how you perceive friendships, will be influenced by your culture, or the type of society you inhabit, and your gender. In Middle Eastern, Asian and Latin American friendships there is an expectation that you will go out of your way to help a friend; indeed, will be self-sacrificing in order to maintain the friendship. Collectivist societies that have an emphasis on groups and communities cooperating together expect close friendship bonds to be established. However, in individualistic societies, such as in North America, you are expected to look out for yourself. Women tend towards more self-disclosure than men and men do not generally view the sharing of intimate details as being necessary in friendships.

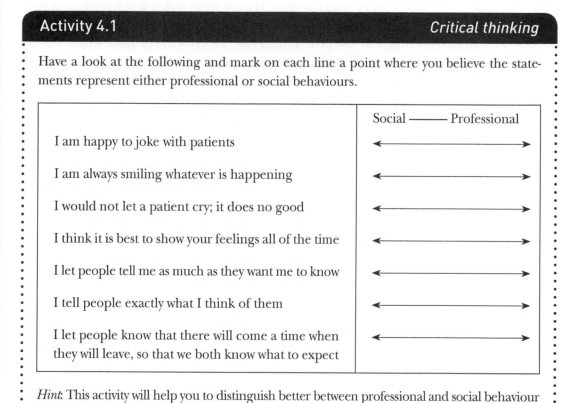

Activity 4.1   *Critical thinking*

Have a look at the following and mark on each line a point where you believe the statements represent either professional or social behaviours.

	Social ——— Professional
I am happy to joke with patients	←———→
I am always smiling whatever is happening	←———→
I would not let a patient cry; it does no good	←———→
I think it is best to show your feelings all of the time	←———→
I let people tell me as much as they want me to know	←———→
I tell people exactly what I think of them	←———→
I let people know that there will come a time when they will leave, so that we both know what to expect	←———→

Hint: This activity will help you to distinguish better between professional and social behaviour and also to reflect critically on aspects of your own behaviour that you may take for granted.

Degrees of intimacy

When talking about intimacy in CIPS, we can be discussing two aspects. One is the physical space between persons in an interaction, which is underpinned by studies in proxemics. The other concerns the degree to which we disclose our inner feelings and thoughts to another, and the extent of self-disclosure required in a relationship to achieve a greater depth of intimacy in knowing and understanding between the partners. Both have relevance to understanding the relative boundaries expected in social and professional relationships.

Proxemics

Hall (1966) pioneered the study of proxemics and identified four spatial distances that also correspond to types of social relationships. They are intimate, personal, social and public.

The four distances can be further divided into close and far phases. The far phase of one level can blend into the close phase of the next level. This will depend on the situation and degrees of comfort felt by individuals and also the shift from one distance to another, either to increase or contract the distance.

The theoretical explanations for these distances are conceptualised in three different ways. The first suggests that individuals hold a buffer of space around them that acts as a protection zone against unwanted attack or touching. As nursing often takes place within this zone, it is important to consider how we move into this close proximity and reduce the sense of threat that this closeness may generate. The second suggests that we strive to maintain equilibrium between varying degrees of intimacy and interpersonal relationships and that we adjust the spatial/relationship ratio accordingly. When the degree of equilibrium that you have chosen is threatened, you may make adjustments, such as avoiding eye contact on a crowded bus or turning away.

The final explanation is derived from responses where individuals find themselves having their expectations of proximity 'violated'. Called the 'expectancy violation theory', it holds that, in these situations, the topic of conversation becomes less important and the relationship comes into focus in its place. Those who violate expected spatial relationships are judged to be less truthful. Yet, if you are perceived positively (that is, of high status or particularly attractive), you will be perceived even more positively if you violate the norm. If, however, you are perceived negatively and you violate the norm, you will be perceived even more negatively. It is a minefield in which nurses have to tread very carefully so as not to violate the expected distance.

A good way to avoid such violation is to seek permission from the patient before carrying out a personal procedure and wait for a response before continuing. This may not be possible in an emergency situation, but it is always advisable to explain to the patient what you are doing and why; even a semi-comatose person can hear a voice and this will enable the patient to be more aware of your actions. Similarly, the tone and pitch of your voice, which should be gently questioning and not commanding, will give the patient reassurance. Informing and negotiating consent to invade a patient's personal space demonstrates respect for the patient's privacy and dignity.

Relationship	Distance
Intimate	0 — 18 inches Close — Far *Very close family and friends*
Casual-Personal	1 ——————— 4 feet Close ——————— Far *Informal conversations with friends and acquaintances*
Social-Consultative	4 ——————————— 12 feet Close ——————————— Far *More impersonal professional transactions*
Public	12 ——————————— 25 feet + Close ——————————— Far *Making speeches and addressing large groups at formal gatherings*

Figure 4.1: Relationships and proxemic distances (adapted from DeVito, 2007)

Self-disclosure

How much do you tell patients about yourself to gain a sense of closeness in your professional relationship and to equalise the reciprocity between the information that you have about them versus the amount they have about you? Creating this balance is seen as a fundamental human need. First, let's consider what we may mean by 'self'. Hargie and Dickson (2004) suggest that there are nine different types of self. To help us understand these many facets, they have conceptualised these types as shown in Table 4.2 (previously discussed in Chapter 2).

Me as	Type of self
I am	Actual self
I would really like to be	Ideal self
I used to be	Past self
I should be	Ought self
A new person	Reconstructed self
I hope to become	Expected self
I'm afraid of becoming	Feared self
I could have been	Missed self
Unwanted by one or more others	Rejected self

Table 4.2: Types of self

Self-disclosure means communicating information about yourself. It may involve information about your values ('taking is not as important as giving love'), beliefs ('I believe that the world is square'), desires ('I would like to fly to the moon and back'), behaviour ('I eat sweets all day long') or self-qualities or characteristics ('I am always happy'). It is a natural part of interpersonal communications and can be verbal or non-verbal. In the former, it can be voluntary, or as a response to information from another person. In the latter, it can manifest itself in the clothes you wear or the way you speak. However it transpires, it can be best seen in the professional nurse–patient relationship as a developing process in which information is exchanged over a period of time, and which changes as the relationship develops from an initial contact to more intimacy, and perhaps to eventual deterioration and closure. It depends very much on the nature of the relationship, whether friend, family, parent, child or professional.

Self-disclosure can be about facts or feelings. When meeting for the first time it is likely that the interaction will be about facts. While you would not be expected to reveal facts about your intimate personal details, you can reveal facts about yourself to equalise the balance, for example how long you have been a nurse or worked on the unit. An acknowledgement to the patient that these are personal questions will help create a recognition of the embarrassment factor.

It is accepted in relationships that there is a gradual progression from lower to higher levels of self-disclosure. However, in the professional nurse–patient relationship it has to be accepted that this is not the case. As deeper levels of disclosure are expected from the patient, the nurse's responsibility is to reassure the patient of the confidentiality related to the assessment and establish levels of trust, respect and confidence in the assessment process so that the patient feels comfortable with what will be an imbalance in reciprocity. A major factor is explaining why the information is needed.

Rules of social engagement

In most social situations, we know how to behave because we have learned the **social rules** that govern or guide the interactions. These have evolved from our experiences of family networks and social groups. Examples are the different words we use to initiate an encounter, such as Hello, Hi, How ya doin'?, What's up? and G'day, which all indicate the appropriate response to follow, which would be Hello, Hi, Jus' fine, Not much and All right, mate.

We have also learned from our regular involvement with activities and events – such as attending lectures, participating in handovers on the unit or having a meal out – the parts we have to play, such as student, staff or friend. This familiarity with social interactions, the expected verbal responses and behaviours gives us a sense of security. We know what to expect, but in new situations, where we might not know the 'rules of engagement' or have an understanding of the shared representations or intersubjective knowledge of what to do, we can feel anxious and isolated. We have to search for clues, observe behaviour patterns or listen to exchanges of information from those already established in the group. This applies to students on their practice learning experiences for the first time and for patients newly admitted or receiving care for the first time.

Research summary

Melia (1984) researched student nurses and found that barriers to socialisation processes were linked to rules. The main thrust of this study was to investigate the occupational socialisation of nursing. Social pressure from staff, and other students, on the wards helped to enforce behaviours that were acceptable to the wards but that did not always put the interests of the patients first. Melia found that, to fit in, students adapted to the new environments by not accepting either the education or service view of acceptable practice. Instead:

Their main concern was to meet the expectations of those with whom they worked, especially those in authority.
(Melia, 1984)

The students thus viewed their training as a series of hurdles to overcome in order to survive. Does this apply to you today or have things changed?

Once the social rules have been learned, people can work and cooperate with a minimum of negotiation. This shared knowledge not only allows us to take for granted social situations, but also makes any kind of adaptation or change to another set of social representations difficult, challenging and, at times, threatening. Not only do we not know how to behave, because we are so accustomed to behaving in a certain manner, but we associate this with a central perception of ourselves that is also challenged. Our notion of who we are and what role we have to play is compromised and causes, for some people, a profound sense of disequilibrium.

Patients can also experience this disequilibrium when they enter healthcare settings. Understanding their perspective and enabling them to have a clear view of what is expected and the role they have to play can reduce anxiety and make communication more effective.

Making the rules explicit rather than implicit can also help. For example, rules forbidding smoking are explicit. Rules for rewarding or punishing behaviours that are perceived to be bad or do not conform to the shared social rules are not so explicit. This is why patients often do not ask questions – because they are wary of breaking a rule and do not know what the sanctions will be if they do not behave in an expected manner.

Goffman (1972) was a seminal investigator of social rules. An example of how rules determine how we behave was better understood from his studies into the social rules around proximity, personal space and gaze, which are socially and implicitly derived. Humans establish rules concerning the distance they feel comfortable with (see the discussion on proxemics earlier in this chapter) and the amount of touching that is acceptable between persons. Gaze is crucial in controlling any invasion of this personal space. Looking into someone's eyes implies an intimacy and a closeness, indicating a desire to know someone well. To avoid a 'forced violation of space' or intimacy we look away. No one usually tells you this rule; instead, you find it out by observing adults as a child or in social situations in adult life, which is why it is both social and implicit. If you get it wrong you would probably experience a rebuff, which is the human way to help individuals to learn the rules.

Because of the complexity of these rules, we sometimes cannot avoid breaking a few. To overcome this Goffman advised minimising the damage by convincing others that we are to be trusted, and that we are competent and worthy. He suggested the following three tactics.

1. Offer an account of why the error happened and give an explanation. This shows that no one is to blame and the error could not be helped – 'I needed to see the other person first because she was just about to go off duty.'

2. Offer an apology that accepts part of the blame. This is also an implicit promise that no harm was intended, that you are aware of the rules and that you can be trusted not to transgress again – 'I'm sorry. I don't know why I did that. I knew immediately afterwards that it was wrong.'

3. Reconstrue the behaviour as one that was not breaking any rules, but was part of another activity – 'I was only joking.'

There are times when the transgression is too serious and these tactics are insufficient. There is a likelihood that sanctions and damage will follow. Gaining support from colleagues is needed to approach the situation in a professional manner with a plan of action to reduce any harm. Explanations and apologies are required to those who feel injured by the mistakes. Avoiding the mistakes will lead to unresolved guilt on the part of the perpetrator and potential repeated incidents of misunderstanding and mistrust.

The emotional context of communicating

Catherine Theodosius (2008) argues that the practice of nursing is emotional labour. In taking this stance, she is encouraging nurses to engage positively with the fact that they cannot avoid the impact of their own emotions, and that of their patients, in nursing practice. Theodosius thus asserts that nurses should strive to make emotional labour therapeutic:

> *Therapeutic emotional labour (TEL) is therefore where the nursing intention is to enable the establishment or maintenance of the interpersonal therapeutic relationship between nurse and patient in order to promote the psychological and emotional wellbeing of the patient in a way that facilitates their movement towards independent health living. TEL is dealing with emotions that are directly concerned with expressions of self-worth and personal identity of both the patient and the nurse, elicited from their interactive relationship . . . TEL may involve giving patients appropriate information on which they can act . . . TEL may involve the nurse encouraging the patient to express and talk about their feelings and concerns while managing their own emotions. It is predicated on the belief that disclosure and discussion of personal and private problems is therapeutic for the patient and, within nursing, is typical of emotional labour represented in the Nightingale ethic. TEL may involve both the nurse and patient accepting the inevitability of death, predicated on the belief that the nurse can facilitate the patient towards as peaceful and dignified a death as possible.*
> (Theodosius, 2008, pp146–147)

Just as for our patients, our emotions are a fundamental part of our personal identity. They can be either pre-programmed (genetic) or learned, and they can be demonstrated in many different ways through our actions and interactions. The phrase 'being emotional' is often used to describe someone who is displaying an overtly emotional reaction to a situation by crying, shouting or being upset. Yet we do not always have to display our emotions to know that we are feeling them. Thus, emotions can be either overt or hidden in the depths of our beings.

Sometimes we are aware of our emotions and sometimes we are not. This all adds up to fascinating, but complicated, phenomena in the human psyche. Emotions are also connected to the positive or negative values we place on objects, persons and situations. Thus, emotions can colour our perceptions of events and add a layer, or filter, to our experiences, which is intended to help us either cope with the exciting, demanding, unfamiliar and unpleasant, or understand the gravity or danger of an experience. Equally, our emotional state can sometimes lead us to impact negatively on our patients, in ways often outside our awareness. This is illustrated in the following case study.

Case study: Two very different nurses

Alistair spends a couple of days in hospital, in order to have a septoplasty procedure carried out on his broken nose. Two student nurses interact with him in relation to routine tasks that have been assigned to them. One is consistently cheerful and friendly with him, and helps him see the funny side of having what feels to him like 300 yards of gauze up his right nostril. From her facial expression, the other nurse always looks miserable and distant. She never speaks with Alistair and appears to him as if she would rather be on another continent. After the cheerful one disappears, presumably at the end of her shift, the occasional ministrations of the miserable-looking one begin to make Alistair wish that she was on another continent.

Theory summary: Emotions

The five emotions most often regarded as being fundamental for human beings are as follows.

Happiness

- This includes joy, contentment, having a warm inner glow, feeling like smiling, feeling a sense of well-being and feeling peace within ourselves. For some, happiness is achieved through pleasure at any cost; for others it is the absence of problems in their lives.
- Happiness is both transient and enduring.
- It can differ over cultures.

Fear and anxiety

- Fear is characterised by being afraid of a threat, danger or harm and by being focused on a particular object or experience.
- Anxiety is a generalised, diffused feeling of being threatened without being able to pinpoint the source of the distress.

(Continued)

(Continued)

- In fear, we can point to the cause; in anxiety we cannot.
- Anxiety is more pervasive and tends to last longer.

Anger

- Anger is often precipitated by frustration at not achieving a goal, suffering injustice or receiving an insult or intentional injury.
- Believing behaviour is unintentional, unavoidable or accidental diminishes anger.
- We are most likely to be angry with people we love than with those we dislike and only slightly towards those we do not know.

Sadness and grief

- Sadness is a mild and relatively brief emotion, whereas grief is a deep and long-lasting period of great sorrow, usually associated with loss.
- Sadness is often caused by making mistakes, being forced to do something against one's judgement, or doing harm to others.
- While it is uncomfortable, sadness has an adaptive quality in that people will try to make redress as a result of sadness.

Disgust

- Disgust is a response to objects or experiences deemed repulsive due to their nature, origin or social history.
- It also has an adaptive function as a motivator to remove ourselves from harm and to reject things that are unsafe.

(Adapted from Sternberg, 2001, p542)

To the emotions above, you could add surprise, guilt (a private sense of culpability) and shame (public humiliation).

Feelings and emotions allow individuals to experience sensitivity and compassion for another, even though they might not fully understand the situation. As has been discussed, the emotions we feel in nursing practice are important, as they are an inevitable part of how we respond and react to the persons in our care and to each other. As illustrated by Alistair's experience in the case study, caring for someone with feeling is qualitatively different from caring for someone in a distant and dispassionate manner. We utilise the information we receive about how a person is responding, whether it is with happiness, sadness or fear, to judge how we manage the interaction and carry out therapeutic interventions. If a person is very fearful of a procedure, the explanation and management of that procedure will require specific tuning to that person's needs. If a person is experiencing significant loss or grief over a change in status or disfigurement from a wound, a nurse will adjust the care plan to take into account these feelings, in order to support and enable adjustment to the change in circumstances. A relative or friend who is angry and behaving aggressively because he or she believes treatment has not been timely or appropriate – often the result of miscommunication or a sense of lack of control – will need sensitive acknowledgement of that person's fears, worries and frustrations by the nurse, and time to assimilate new information.

Balancing emotions

Our aim in life is to have a healthy balance of emotional experiences. This involves letting go of feelings that are damaging, or restricting adjustments to new situations, and searching for new ways of dealing with situations that provoke emotional responses. This is complicated when individuals are unable to express their emotions, which may in turn be a function of not knowing what emotions they are feeling due to confusion, unusual circumstances or changes in the status quo. Alternatively, people may know what they are feeling but not understand why, or may be experiencing conflicting emotions about the same situation. The nurse's role in these circumstances is to help patients clarify and identify their feelings with the aim of enabling a healthy expression or outlet for the feelings. The best way to do this is to:

- understand the underlying reasons that have provoked the emotional response;
- allow the person to tell his or her story;
- identify an emotion that is being labelled in the story, for example, 'It must be frightening not to understand what is happening to your body right now';
- ask to help in a non-reactive way, which demonstrates caring by helping to obtain the needed information and validate the fears;
- identify if the person needs a break from the intensity of the situation, for example by arranging to come back later to talk over concerns again.

All these actions are key to developing an understanding and appreciation of the emotional context of a situation from the patient's perspective.

Harmful emotional expression

Emotions can be harmful when they block adjusting to new situations, get out of control or affect another person by reducing self-esteem. Unresolved feelings can lead to communication misunderstandings in which needs are not perceived to be met. Feelings perceived to be unacceptable can be hidden behind a mask of calm or rationality. Repressed feelings can be expressed with an excessive intensity that is disproportionate to the situation. Consequently, communication and relationships can be distorted by misperceptions created through emotions that are unexpressed, over-expressed or inappropriately expressed. Therefore, the feelings about the content of an interaction have to be balanced with the feelings about what is happening to the self or others in any situation (Hargie, 2006).

. . . .

Case study: Coping with bereavement

Layla, a first-year student nurse, begins a practice learning experience on a ward where there are elderly patients. She is suffering from unresolved grief over the recent death of her beloved grandmother. The ward staff notice that she is finding it difficult to interact with the elderly women on the ward. A staff nurse, who is her mentor, sensitively talks with her about this. When she finds out the reason behind the student's difficulty, she also hears that Layla has carried her grief alone, without sharing her feelings with anyone. Layla agrees to talk with her sisters and parents about how she is feeling, and within a couple of weeks she is able to interact positively with the elderly women on the ward.

. . . .

Barriers to communication and interpersonal relationships

Before considering the barriers, it is relevant to review the aims of communication and initiating relationships in the healthcare context. From your reading in this book, we hope you will have gathered your own precepts to guide you towards effective interactions; however, here are a few that we hope you have included in your list:

- establishing a trusting and respectful relationship;
- transmitting and sharing information;
- exchanging ideas and understanding perceptions;
- creating a platform for renewed understanding;
- enhancing understanding of attitudes, ideas and beliefs;
- achieving mutually acceptable goals for discourse, interventions and therapy.

An essential ingredient for interactions to be effective is for meanings to be shared and understood. To do this, meanings have to be checked and an awareness created to intercept blocks to communication that can arise from the many differences in individuals, such as authority, power, language, ability and disability, personality, background, gender, health, age, race and socioeconomic group.

Meaning

It is believed that genuine communication can only be achieved if barriers are identified and worked through. Exploring the meaning, which is an active process created between participants in an interaction between source and receiver, speaker and listener, writer and reader, can help identify some of those barriers. Meaning is not only dependent on messages but also on the interaction between the messages and the thoughts and feelings within those messages. Consequently, meaning is not just 'received'; it is constructed or built up from messages that are received and combined with social and cultural perspectives, for example beliefs, attitudes and values.

It is not just the words that people use; it is the meaning or interpretation that each person gives to the words that construct the meaning. If the understanding of the meaning is shared, there is less likely to be a barrier to communication.

Activity 4.3   *Reflection*

Below are five topical concepts and a potential rating descriptor. Consider each concept and place your own descriptor/word that represents the meaning you have for that concept in the graded column that represents your strength of feeling along a continuum of good to bad. Compare your sense of meanings with a peer.

Concept	Good 1	2	3	4	Bad 5
Abortion					
Terrorism					
Schooling					
Death penalty					
Euthanasia					

An added challenge is that no two individuals are likely to derive exactly the same meaning and, because people change their views and ideas about life, it is not always possible to predict accurately another's sense of meaning. Indeed, your own meanings may change from one day to the next depending on your experiences. To refine this process as much as possible, verify the perception you have of another's meanings by asking probing questions, echoing what you perceive to be the other's feelings or thoughts, and seeking elaboration or clarification. In general, practise the communication skills we have discussed in this book. Ultimately, it is wise not to assume that the meaning you attribute to phenomena, actions, situations, behaviours and emotional responses will correspond with someone else's.

Motivation towards being healthy

One barrier that may impede the nurse–patient relationship is reluctance by the patient to follow health advice. This is a barrier associated with individuals' beliefs about the cause of their illness or their health and well-being. Advising patients to follow treatment regimes or adopt different lifestyle choices to maintain or improve their health requires a detailed understanding of how health beliefs are constructed. It requires a concentrated form of communication that builds upon the strategies already presented, but that may be content-specific, in contrast to a free-flowing therapeutic style. This is because the nurse is deliberately including information for the patient to hear and understand, and which has consequences for the future health of the patient. There is also a clearer expectation of the outcome, which is that the patient will follow a medication regime, or undertake specific daily activities that may require learning a different or new set of skills.

There are several models in the literature that guide this process. Role performance models evaluate functioning and successful outcomes as benchmarks of achievement in adopting new health behaviours. Adaptive models consider self-care approaches to alteration in behaviours. Self-fulfilment has also been incorporated into these models, borrowed from Maslow's hierarchy of needs and the **eudaemonistic** model proposed by Smith (1987). Smith proposed that health was made up of four dimensions: (1) the absence of disease; (2) the ability to function according to the expectations of the society in which a person lives; (3) the ability to adjust and change according to circumstances; and (4) the ability to realise one's potential. This last dimension is similar to the pinnacle of Maslow's (1943) model of a hierarchy of human needs, which represents personal growth and fulfilment or, in the words of Maslow, *self-actualization*. In the hierarchy, Maslow proposed five levels, often reproduced in the form of a triangle. The base of the triangle represents fundamental human needs, deemed to be physiological or biological needs. Above this are safety and security, followed by love and friendship, and above this self-esteem. Maslow's theory suggests that the most basic needs must be met before higher-level needs can be achieved. Successful achievement of these is acquired through the hierarchy based upon an individual's motivation to achieve the highest level of human need.

Conflict

It may be difficult to accept, but it is widely agreed by many writers that there are times in every relationship when those involved will agree to differ, and the healthcare context is no exception. Misunderstandings arise when conflict is experienced and it is assumed that there is something wrong with the situation or that the relationship is in jeopardy or damaged. A difference of opinion is not a conflict; it is where two sets of creative thought or ideas differ. The situation that becomes misunderstood or develops into an aggressive outburst is one where the misunderstandings have expanded to include personal egos, lack of trust and emotional perceptions that distort the relativity of the situation. The role of the nurse in situations of conflict is to be aware of the dynamics and the skills required for resolution.

Conflict can serve as an alarm to indicate that a relationship needs closer attention. It sometimes offers an opportunity to clarify differences of opinion and in a therapeutic relationship may be necessary to work towards achieving a different set of behaviours or responses from the patient. The disadvantages of conflict are increasing negativity, hurting others and depleting energy that is needed for other emotional tasks. The positive effects are that it can lead to a closer examination of issues that are rearing up in a relationship or group. Examining the problems and finding solutions to the conflict can be a way of mending bridges and strengthening relationships. Nonetheless, experiencing conflict can be disquieting and uncomfortable, giving rise to feelings that can be challenging or in opposition to closely held beliefs or values.

The first step in conflict resolution is to analyse the situation. Arnold and Boggs (2007) state that the things to consider are:

- previous experiences with conflict situations;
- the degree to which the conflict is acceptable;
- the intensity of the feeling it arouses;
- the physical, cognitive and emotional health or stamina of the persons involved;

- the subjective interpretation of the event or conflict;
- the consequences.

Conflict can become manageable when the causes, sources and issues underpinning the conflict are clearly articulated by the parties involved. This needs time and the use of non-judgemental listening skills to collect the stories. By drawing out hidden feelings or repressed ideas that otherwise may not have been known, barriers to communication can be identified and resolved.

One of the most common responses to conflict is anger. Anger is one of our fundamental emotions, as mentioned above. It originates in a part of the brain called the amygdala, which is responsible for thought and judgements. The anger response is intended to identify threats and prepare our bodies for attack. This is a rapid response that is very necessary in life-threatening situations; however, it does not always give us time to think about appropriate responses or the consequences of our actions.

Theory summary: Aggressive behaviour

The human response to conflict is defensive, and defensive behaviour can also be aggressive.

There are three forms of aggressive behaviour: aggressive, passive and passive-aggressive.

- The aggressive response is to deflect the attack through attacking back at a personal level, or blaming, which generates feelings in the other person of anger and resentment.
- The passive response is self-preservation by not engaging in, or by not wishing to resolve, the conflict. This generates feelings of frustration and loss of respect.
- The passive-aggressive response is where, on the surface, a person appears to be agreeing to plans and arrangements that are made, but in reality is not engaging with the activities designed to solve the problems. There can be verbal agreement at the same time as sabotaging or discrediting activities undertaken by the passive-aggressor, which leads to confusion and mistrust.

Activity 4.4   *Team working*

With a group of peers, identify the sources of conflict that you have witnessed in the clinical areas you have experienced so far. Separate out those situations that involved staff to staff, staff to patients, patients to staff, and patient to patient. Analyse these situations to identify common features of the causes of conflict.

What examples have you witnessed of good conflict management? Compare these with poorly managed examples.

Hint: This activity is aimed at helping you start to develop your skills in conflict recognition and conflict management. Often conflicts are allowed to fester and grow in healthcare environments, usually to the detriment of patient and client care.

The second step in conflict resolution is to identify the potential solutions to the problems or issues that are causing the conflict. Key elements for any professional involved in a conflict situation are to remember that the rights of the individuals involved are to be respected and to behave in an assertive manner. Assertiveness needs to be learned and the websites listed at the end of the chapter will provide you with some resources to work through. If you are going to set up a meeting to resolve conflict, Arnold and Boggs (2007) suggest that you will need to consider the following.

- *Prepare for the encounter.* Be clear about the purpose, the major points to discuss and whether the information you have is complete and can be shared. Give careful consideration to the language used and the choice of words so that messages are clear and unambiguous.

- *Organise your information* and consult with another to validate your approach, preferably someone who is objective. Rehearse.

- *Manage your own anxiety.* Use breathing and relaxation techniques to calm you. Think of a mantra to reinforce your commitment to your rights.

- *Time the encounter.* Judge when parties will be receptive, allow time for discussion and expressions of choice and be prepared to listen.

- *Take one issue at a time* and focus on the present. Break the problem down into small units or steps and allow time for clarification. If one small area can be resolved, this can lead to further resolutions.

- *Request a change* in behaviour or response. Assess the level of readiness and take into consideration maturity, culture, values and life factors.

- *Evaluate the conflict resolution.* It may take more time; small goals can be achieved first. Aim for a climate of openness and future communication.

Taking steps to solve problems and reduce conflict requires skilled handling and can be achieved through observation and practice in role play.

Chapter summary

In this chapter we have explored relationship boundaries between professional relationships and friendships/kinships. We have also looked at relevant research and the implications of intimacy and proximity. Emotions, and how they need to be balanced to achieve effective communication outcomes, have been discussed and you should now understand the construction of meaning and how this underpins communication messages. We have stressed the importance of interpreting meanings to clarify understanding and perceptions of events, and you should have learned how motivation factors can affect health messages, and how to identify the benefits and barriers to achieving health-promoting communications. We have also explained how conflicts can arise and how they should be handled in healthcare settings.

Further reading

Arnold, E and Boggs, KU (2015) *Interpersonal Relationships: Professional communication skills for nurses,* 7th edn. Philadelphia, PA: WB Saunders.

This is a useful book that further clarifies some of the issues raised in this text.

Srof, BJ and Velsor-Friedrich, B (2006) Health promotion in adolescents: a review of Pender's health promotion model. *Nursing Science Quarterly,* 19(4): 366–373.

Theodosius, C (2008) *Emotional Labour in Health Care: The unmanaged heart of nursing.* London: Routledge.

This book is an excellent primer on the role of emotion in the work of nursing, including the practice of CIPS.

Useful websites

www.businessballs.com/self-confidence-assertiveness.htm

This website has information on assertiveness training.

www.mentalhelp.net/poc/center_index.php?id=116&cn=116

This site about anger management has many resources on explaining the physiology and psychology of anger as well as techniques for managing angry outbursts.

Chapter 5
The learning and educational context of communication and interpersonal skills

NMC Standards for Pre-registration Nursing Education

This chapter will address the following competencies:

Domain 2: Communication and interpersonal skills

2. All nurses must use a range of communication skills and technologies to support person-centred care and enhance quality and safety. They must ensure people receive all the information they need in a language and manner that allows them to make informed choices and share decision-making. They must recognise when language interpretation or other communication support is needed and know how to obtain it.

6. All nurses must take every opportunity to encourage health-promoting behaviour through education, role modelling and effective communication.

7. All nurses must maintain accurate, clear and complete records, including the use of electronic formats, using appropriate and plain language.

NMC Essential Skills Clusters

This chapter will address the following ESCs:

Cluster: Care, compassion and communication

6. People can trust the newly registered graduate nurse to engage therapeutically and actively listen to their needs and concerns, responding using skills that are helpful, providing information that is clear, accurate, meaningful and free from jargon.

By the first progression point:

1. Communicates effectively both orally and in writing, so that the meaning is always clear.

By the second progression point:

6. Uses strategies to enhance communication and remove barriers to effective communication, minimising risk to people from lack of poor communication.

Introduction

You will have many learning goals in your time as a student and this chapter will guide you in achieving these through enhanced CIPS. So far in this book we have been focusing on CIPS for your role as a professional. In this chapter we will be focusing on how CIPS can support you and your individual learning pathway – now and throughout your career. The way we will do this is to look at a spectrum of your role as learner through to educator and eventually your own continuing learning needs as a lifelong learner (Figure 5.1).

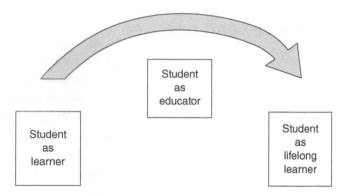

Figure 5.1: Spectrum of learner, educator and lifelong learner

This chapter will examine each of the three stages in the spectrum, beginning with a discussion on you as a student and learner. We will explore some of the issues related to the integration of theory and practice. This leads us to discuss how learning should be realistic and relevant to your practice and learning needs. One way to achieve this is through experiential learning techniques, which we will explore through a model. Learning through experience is regarded as learning by doing, rather than by listening to others or reading. This form of learning involves active, rather than passive, learning through interactions, self-awareness, expression, flexibility and reciprocity, and with relevance or meaning. All these characteristics are present in CIPS as they are very much related to how you behave in interpersonal situations. Consequently, learning *through* experience (which refers to deliberately planned learning experiences) and learning *from* experience (which refers to past experiences to gain new insights) are two highly relevant learning approaches in CIPS.

Following this, a framework for levels of academic qualifications is presented with a discussion on how this links to practice. The skills gained from examining this framework will enable you to operate more effectively within complex care environments for decision making, and will facilitate problem-solving, critical thinking and reflective capacities. We have drawn links to the assessment of practice requirements to enable you to have a clearer idea of how to gain proficiency in skills. We have also included sections on reflective writing, learning styles and the characteristics of a skilled performance, which will help you complete your practice learning assessments and put CIPS into practice.

There are many different contexts in which students can act as educators among colleagues and with patients, in order to give instruction or guidance on health promotion or health education perspectives. Guidelines for improving communication in these settings are provided, along with a description of the professional standards required in these circumstances.

The final section of the chapter looks to the future and considers the role of a student in formulating a frame of mind to include lifelong learning. We look at the importance of skills from a health policy perspective and consider the extended scope of practice through career trajectories and forward thinking.

The student as learner

Integration of theory and practice

One of the constant dilemmas for nursing students during their studies is the need to integrate theories learned in the classroom with the practice of nursing performed in clinical, real-world situations. This is no easier with CIPS, which can seem so obvious and yet, as this book demonstrates, are not just simple skill sets to be learned in a rote fashion. We all have CIPS abilities and what has to be achieved during studies is enhancing, improving and making more effective these skills in healthcare settings. We have already explored some theories in this book and have attempted to use practical exercises to demonstrate how the theory can be applied. Judging how meaningful these are and how they can be applied to good effect helps with the integration of theory with practice. But it may not be enough.

The NMC *Standards for Pre-registration Nursing Education* (2010) assert that practice, integrated with theory, needs to be evidence-based, thus safe. In Chapter 2, we explored the importance of integrating theory with practice and the relationship to research that provides the evidence for safe practice. As with any practice-based skill, practice makes perfect and this applies equally to CIPS. Practising using the skills by working with models in an environment that is safe, exactly in the same way that you might practise inserting a nasogastric tube, is as essential as rehearsing practical skills. The difference may be the self-consciousness or self-awareness you may have as you say words that are unfamiliar or use phrases that, at first, sound false and stilted. The conditions you need in order to practise are therefore important.

Activity 5.1	*Reflection*

What are the ideal conditions that you need in order to practise a new communication or interpersonal skill?

Do you need to be alone and in front of a mirror? Or do you need to be with a close friend, or in a group? Each of these situations can pose different levels of complexity in communication, how you use your interpersonal skills and the feedback you will get on the effectiveness of your skills.

Hint: This activity will help you increase your awareness of your CIPS learning style. It will help you learn about practice situations that inhibit you, compared with those in which you feel more relaxed. Generally, it is good to proceed from relaxed to increasingly inhibiting situations.

Disconcertingly, there is continuing evidence that final-year nursing students and newly qualified nurses have difficulty sustaining the values and ideals they gained during their training (Jasper, 1996; Maben et al., 2006, 2007a). Maben et al. (2006) found that, while nurses had gained a strong set of values during their programmes of study, there were professional and organisational factors that prevented them from taking their ideas into practice. The study felt that this had serious consequences for the integration of theory with practice, as the need to obey covert rules, lack of support and poor role models inhibited newly qualified nurses in carrying out their ideas of evidenced-based practice and appropriate standards of care. There were additional demands, such as time pressures, constraints on roles – that is, boundaries and opportunities – shortages of staff and work overload. By practising and applying the ideas, concepts and theories (the summaries of how these concepts are organised) during and beyond your course, you will be working towards closing the theory–practice gap.

Learning for reality

Eve Bendall (1976) was one of the first nurse researchers to study the theory–practice gap. In her seminal work on how students learn clinical skills, which she called learning for reality, she found, when observing students in practice and comparing this with what they wrote, that they described one thing in writing and then did something completely different in practice. The classroom assumption was that a written description by a student nurse would be sufficient evidence to judge that the nurse was competent to carry out care for specific patient conditions. Her study found the assumption to be false and was pivotal in formulating the practice-based curriculum that nurses experience today.

Today's nurses are deemed to be more patient-focused and more effective in social interaction. This is credited to the inclusion of theoretical concepts drawn from the social sciences into nursing care. These are integrated into theoretical models of nursing specifically designed to guide care, yet nursing remains a practice-based profession requiring the demonstration of skills proficiencies. Over time, nursing skills have expanded from purely physical activities with, for example, visual, auditory, verbal, tactile, kinaesthetic and organisational factors, to include those underpinned by the social sciences, including, for example, the psychological, social, interactive, interpretive and conceptual factors we are exploring in this book (Bendall, 2006).

There are different views about how best to enable nurses to learn practical skills. One view is that principles should be taught early in the course, so that they can then be taken into practice settings, and applied and practised in different situations until competency is reached. In this approach, evidence-based care is taken to the practice area and carried out in vivo – in the living and real environment. The tasks are supervised by a qualified mentor and then assessed.

Another view is for students to observe care being delivered and for the elements of nursing care in any one situation to be identified by the students. So, for example, in a ward or community setting, the nurse carries out different actions with and for the patients. The task of the student is to make note of these activities and assemble these into a whole picture of care that is required for that particular setting. Once assembled, students follow up the tasks to discover whether there is evidence underpinning the activities, discriminate between the essential and unessential elements and determine if there are sequences or levels of ordering in the elements to enable them to apply the activities when they are required to do so without supervision. This is a more complex method, but is more detailed, and requires mentors to establish whether or not students have identified the relevant parts of the whole, their relative significance and appropriateness in the situation.

Each of these approaches has advantages. The first is that students are prepared with ideas and strategies before they enter the practice setting. Many students find this comforting, as they do not wish to be seen as incompetent when they find themselves working with patients. It also enables students to feel confident about a situation that has the potential to undermine their confidence. The second is based on the **gestalt** idea that all experiences are based on the sum of the individual parts and that, by examining the parts, a whole can be assembled with better understanding of how the parts interact. The term 'gestalt' is derived from the German term meaning 'pattern' or 'configuration' and this enables learning. The patterns are thought to stand out from the background against which they are seen, giving rise to the concepts of figure and ground in perceiving phenomena.

Experiential learning

A third approach to practice learning is through experiential learning. This is where individuals go through a process of experiencing, reflecting, thinking and acting. Kolb and Fry (1975) proposed this theory, which claims that experiencing a phenomenon leads to observations and reflections. They believed that these activities form a cycle of activities that make up a four-stage learning cycle. Feeling in this context does not describe an emotional experience, although that may contribute to the experience. Feeling is intended to mean a perceived physical or mental sensation. It could also relate to a particular impression, appearance, effect or atmosphere sensed from something, such as a feeling of abandonment about a building. We cannot also rule out that feeling can relate to an instinctive awareness or presentiment of something, such as a prediction that someone will be disappointed with some news. A simple model of these activities is represented in Figure 5.2.

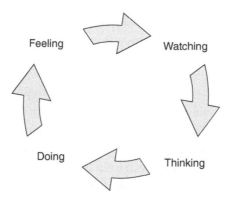

Figure 5.2: A simplistic model of Kolb and Fry's experiential learning theory

Kolb and Fry originally based this model on their work with groups. The model has been further adapted to include the processes of reviewing data and information that will happen during thinking about the experience. The next stage is to puzzle out or give some meaning to the experience. This is then added to the ideas that will influence any further experiences or responses to situations (Figure 5.3). The main premise is that we all have an intrinsic tendency to draw upon our experiences of the world we live in. This helps us to improve our knowledge of what happens to us, and to formulate our opinions and extend our range of skills and knowledge.

We are constantly taking in information through our senses and digesting this information as we experience events, which means that we are never completely in static situations. Even those folk who give the appearance of 'switching off' are still receiving some information, although they wish to give the impression that they are not dealing with it for one reason or another, such as tiredness, dislike of a situation or, in the case of illness, pain and discomfort. They are deliberately turning off that engagement switch or, more likely, tuning down.

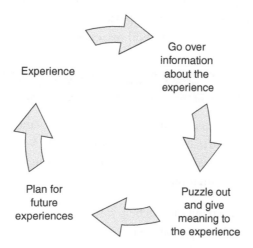

Figure 5.3: Experiential learning cycle

Using experience to guide our actions and beliefs does, however, present its challenges. If our current reactions are based solely on previous experiences, this will inhibit our future learning. While our previous experiences may stand us in good stead in most situations, they may also not always provide us with sufficient solutions to the problems we have to solve. We are never in a position where our accrued experiences will prepare us sufficiently for the next challenge, whatever that may be. Thus, wisdom based only on past experience is limited. We need to be open to learn from new and novel situations.

Our decisions to base our actions on previous experiences may also be founded on assumptions, whether 'true' or 'false', and either our conscious or unconscious assimilation of ideas. It is the stage of the cycle where we ascribe meaning to events and experiences. By interpreting the experiences, and attempting to understand why something is happening, we use different strategies to give an event meaning. Meaning can be drawn from the symbolism of an event – such as a memorial service, which signifies sadness. Or it can be drawn from the notion of what the significance or magnitude of an event represents to someone. Some experiences will therefore have more significance to some than to others, such as attending the memorial service of one's spouse or partner. Meaning can also be drawn from a moral or psychological sense of purpose. For example, 'If I work hard and qualify as a nurse, I'll be able to make an important contribution to the world.'

We rely on our previous experiences to guide our responses but do not necessarily learn from, or adjust, our responses to improve how we react in situations. Most of the time we place our memories of experiences in 'cold storage' or classify them as 'unfinished business', to be returned to when we have enough psychological energy. This explanation can help us understand why some people never learn from experience, because they never return to the cold storage of their memories. To enable us to learn from those experiences we need to combine 'here and now' learning and reflection (see Siviter and Stevens (2004) for practical guidance on surviving as a student nurse).

This is the essence of experiential learning. It is not just learning to do something differently next time, but is more about actively engaging in an analysis and reflection on what has been learned, how it compares with previous learning and how this accumulative store of learning can be built upon further to improve skills and knowledge. This is so relevant when learning about CIPS. You will have already stored up many experiences of your own and will have also refined some of your interpersonal skills as a result of those experiences.

Activity 5.2 *Reflection*

Take a moment to think about a communication misunderstanding that you have experienced. Now consider what you learned from that experience. What was your interpretation of it? How would you improve your communication of information in that experience the next time you face a similar situation?

Hint: This activity, if practised regularly, will help you engage in the experiential learning cycle described in Figure 5.3, and thus prepare you better for future communication encounters.

In nursing, students are given time to learn in practice under the guidance of mentors or experienced healthcare practitioners. In the same way that you learn to carry out a physical procedure, it is important first to observe communication and interpersonal interactions. You can then practise under supervision and be prepared to undertake communication of information on your own. At each stage of the process, you will continue to learn and you will need to create opportunities to review what you are learning, clarify what you have learned from past experiences and think about future experiences to extend your skills. So that you can also gain optimally from these experiences, it is important to know when you are learning by experience as distinct from learning from experience.

Learning by experience is more or less an unconscious process. It is a realisation after the experience that we have learned something significant. These experiences are gained through the reality of professional life, varying and unpredictable demands and changing circumstances. An example of this is that we can often be so preoccupied with getting something right that, when we forget to try and we get it right, there is a sudden integration of knowledge and surprise that the skill can be mastered after all.

To get the most out of these experiences, you need to hone your skills of attention to both external events and what you are experiencing internally. Internal processes include noticing your thoughts, intuitions, emotions, bodily sensations, intentions for yourself and others, needs, what you are doing, how you are doing it and how all this relates together (Figure 5.4).

There is a balance to be struck between being immersed in an experience and totally absorbed by it, and being a witness. So that you can learn from the experience, ask yourself the following questions.

- What am I thinking, feeling or noticing now that describes this situation?
- Am I experiencing any tensions in my body?
- What am I imagining, assuming or presuming?

To help you become more aware, begin to verbalise your thoughts and feelings about experiences to fellow students or mentors.

Learning from experience is a more deliberate and conscious experience. The intention is not just to experience the 'here and now', but to devise future actions based on the reflection and evaluation of events.

Using the experiential learning cycle (look back at Figure 5.3) requires time for thinking and reflection. Some of this goes on informally in social groups or at the end of a shift with groups of peers. The more aware we become of our feelings and intuitions about experiences and the comparison of these reflections on both inner and outer experiences, the more objective our memories of the experiences will be. By practising use of the experiential cycle, students can begin to work through the stages without checking where they are at each stage. Thus, the process of reflection becomes integrated as an evaluative process for refining skills. This will serve to enhance the reflections and learning through experience to greater effect.

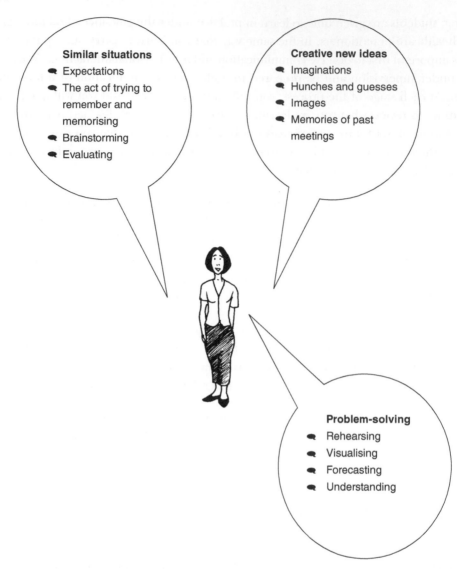

Figure 5.4: Examples of thoughts and intuitions

Assessment of practice in portfolios

Bearing in mind that you need to demonstrate a wide range of thinking skills alongside your development of practice skills, there remains the thorny issue of how both theory (which is an intellectual activity related to your thinking skills) and practice can be captured in one place to demonstrate the achievement of competence. One method is by using portfolios of evidence. Since the early 1990s, portfolios were used to capture evidence of nursing students' learning in practice. Over the years, these have been consistently developed and improved from initially being bulky repositories for sheaves of paper to slimmer versions providing a succinct method for collating evidence. They have now become an integral part of the majority of nursing education programmes (see Reed and Standing (2011) for further guidance).

Reflective writing

It is generally agreed that **reflective writing** is considered the key to assessment by portfolio. This is because it provides evidence of the development of skills and can demonstrate increasing clinical competence over a period of time. We would expect to see development over time as you cannot expect to be competent straight away. Smith (1997) found some evidence that reflection assisted the integration of practice experience with academic knowledge. Development over time was also another feature of this study. However, in a study by Smith and Jack (2005), students were asked if reflection was a meaningful activity and no consensus of opinion was reached. The authors did find that the students' learning style was highly pertinent to their perception of the usefulness of reflection (Howatson-Jones, 2013).

Learning styles

There are several theories on learning styles and these have been reviewed by Coffield et al. (2004). The majority focus on three or four main attributes. Two of the most widely used are the learning-style inventories of Kolb (2000) (whose experiential learning theory we examined earlier in this chapter) and of Honey and Mumford (1992). Both of these versions can easily be found on the internet for you to test out yourself (see useful websites at the end of the chapter). Essentially, Kolb's inventory suggests that we each have a preference for one of four styles: concrete experience (feeling), reflective observation (watching), abstract conceptualisation (thinking) and active experimentation (doing). These are clustered into two continua with conflicting axes: feeling and thinking versus watching and doing. Kolb believes that we choose to learn by grasping at an experience to transform it into something that is meaningful and useful. Our learning styles are therefore a product of either preferring to watch and do, or think and feel.

Honey and Mumford, however, believe there are also four dimensions to learning styles. They describe these as characteristics and divide people into activists, who learn by doing; reflectors, who stand back and observe first; theorists, who prefer to adapt and integrate experiences into a conceptual whole or framework; and pragmatists, who, while on the lookout for new ideas, will only adopt ideas if they have a practical benefit. There are some similarities between Kolb's and Honey and Mumford's approaches to learning styles, but you may want to ponder over which is your preferred style. This might be a good idea, as the research suggests that those students who could relate to the tasks through meaningful reflection were best able to utilise the experience of portfolio learning and the impact that reflection could have on their learning.

Identifying your preferred learning style will help you recognise the work you will need to do on other areas of the dimensions described above, in order to become more reflective. If, for example, you recognise that you are primarily a pragmatist or 'doing' learner, you may wish to work on your capacity for observing, thinking and feeling. Such practice should result in an improvement in your approach to reflection as a learning strategy and in you having a more positive outlook towards this form of learning. This is borne out by a study of pre-clinical medical students undertaken by Rees and Sheard (2004), who found that students who were more positive about reflective portfolios were more likely to rate their reflection skills as good, achieve higher marks for their portfolios and have more confidence in building future portfolios.

Research summary: Reflection in nursing practice

If you are a person who finds reflection difficult and who has a tendency to pragmatism and learning only for reality, you may want to consider the research of Teekman (2000) on exploring reflection in nursing practice using a sense-making approach. He searched for sense-making activities in a group of qualified nurses to examine how they made sense of situations as well as their thought processes. He found that reflective thinking was apparent in moments of doubt and perplexity, categorising perceptions, framing and self-questioning to gain sense and understanding of what was happening in situations.

You may be using reflective thinking without realising if you have ever had a mental tussle over what to do in a difficult situation. You now need to use those same thinking activities and apply them to all situations. This will help you delve deeper into your levels of learning and improve your analytical abilities. In the sense-making theory utilised in Teekman's research, situations are identified as the inexplicable inconsistencies of human experience that are influenced by culture, social organisation and individual perception. There is then a gap where individuals are stopped in their tracks (that is, in a state of discontinuity), where routine thinking is no longer applicable and where new constructions or solutions are required in order to create a personal sense of the situation. 'Uses' is the last stage of the activity, where the individual puts the new thinking into practical use.

Skilled performance

While you may now realise that experiential learning, reflective writing and your preferred learning style may influence how you achieve your learning goals in the assessment of your practice, you will want to know what makes a skilled performance stand out when practice is being assessed. Some essential characteristics are outlined in Table 5.1.

Accuracy	Skill executed with precision
Speed	Movements are swift and confident
Efficiency	Movements are economical, with the ability to draw upon additional movement when required
Timing	Timing is accurate and the sequential order is correct
Consistency	Results are consistent, and repeated successfully on different occasions
Anticipation	Can anticipate events very quickly and respond accordingly
Adaptability	Can adapt the skill to current circumstances
Perception	Can obtain maximum information from a minimum of cues

Table 5.1: Essential characteristics of skilled performance

As mentioned before, any skill has to be practised before it is learned. The more you practise your communication skills with colleagues and friends, and think about the different situations that require different responses, the more it will help you refine your skills and improve your confidence. You are also advised to hone your observational skills and make notes of situations in, for example, the classroom, waiting rooms, clinics and in practice. Evaluate these interactions and conjure up scenarios where you would improve your skills. By developing the skills of observation and analysis, inviting feedback and considering the context in which nursing practice takes place, your critical reflection skills will also develop and you will avoid any negatively framed, overly introspective analysis.

The student as educator

You may only regard yourself as a student who is there to learn rather than teach. But we would propose that there will be opportunities when you will find yourself giving an explanation, directions, instructions or a presentation, or untangling a misunderstanding, and you will be – in effect – teaching another person some aspect of healthcare (Arnold and Boggs, 2007). This could be teaching a fellow student either in the practice setting or in the classroom, explaining to patients or clients about their health or disease, giving advice on promoting healthy wellbeing or even talking to qualified staff if you are presenting a project you have undertaken as part of your studies. There are many self-help texts around to guide you with teaching skills, which is why in this chapter we will be concentrating on how you can communicate clearly, using interpersonal skills effectively to transmit information when you act as an educator (Quinn and Hughes, 2007).

Seven top health communication skills

Because there are so many factors affecting communication between healthcare professionals, and between those professionals and patients or clients, it is difficult to refine the competencies into a 'laundry list'. However, seven top health communication skills have been distilled from different research studies and are outlined briefly here. These should be read with interprofessional communication (communication between yourself and other healthcare professionals) in mind, as well as communication between yourself and your nursing colleagues, and between yourself and your colleagues and patients. The skill tips that follow will also help you in your role as *advocate* between patients and other nursing and healthcare staff. As a student nurse, you may find yourself spending more time with patients, and getting to know them better, than with qualified nursing and other healthcare staff. As a result, there may be times when it will be helpful for you to represent the views and situation of patients to your colleagues.

1. Giving accurate and sufficient feedback

Feedback is a message sent back to the message sender to give reassurance that the message has been received and understood. For example, it is reassuring for patients or clients to receive feedback that they have been understood, or for you to receive reassurance from them that they have understood you. Also, do not be afraid to give positive feedback to colleagues to encourage further good performance. Too often, healthcare staff believe themselves to be continually caught up in punishment dialogues, with their positive contributions to their jobs ignored.

If you are uncertain whether something has been clearly understood by your nursing, medical or other healthcare colleagues, ask for confirmation, or ask if any further explanation is required. Alternatively, if you see an inaccuracy in performance, or poor performance, do not be afraid to bring this to the attention of qualified staff.

Non-verbal feedback is equally important, as it registers reactions to what has been said in, for example, facial expressions such as surprise, boredom or hostility. Non-verbal behaviour needs to be in synchrony with verbal messages, to minimise the risk of 'double' or conflicting messages. As described in the previous chapter, our non-verbal behaviour can sometimes give away our emotions and preoccupations when we are least aware of this, no matter what we say verbally, often to the detriment of our relationships with our patients or colleagues. Even apparently innocuous behaviours, such as leaving the room or remaining silent, are non-verbal communications that may give negative signals to, or alienate, those we care for or those we work with.

2. Listening attentively

This means actively attending to what is being said and how it is being said. It is listening without making judgements or letting your own perceptions act as a barrier to what is being said by the other person. It requires giving signals that you are actively listening by using appropriate prompts, such as 'mmm', 'I see', 'how interesting' or 'OK', and non-verbal prompts, such as nodding and smiling, and also giving feedback to show that you understand what is being said or conveyed. Such *active listening* indicates that you are working hard to understand the other person, and enables trusting relationships, rapport, mutual interest and understanding.

Activity 5.3   *Communication*

Arrange two chairs back to back. Have a friend sit on one chair and yourself on the other. Have the friend tell you about a journey s/he has just taken. Let him or her speak for a couple of minutes. Do not interrupt your friend or ask any questions. When your friend has stopped, recount to him/her what s/he told you. Then place the chairs facing each other. Sit opposite your friend and ask him or her to tell you about his or her day at work for two minutes. Again, do not interrupt or ask questions. When s/he has finished, relate back to him or her what s/he has recounted to you.

Compare the two experiences from two points.

- How did it feel to listen and not speak?
- Did you remember more from the first or the second task about the events?

Hint: What pass for 'normal' social exchanges are often 'duologues' rather than dialogues, with one person waiting for the other to stop talking so that s/he can start talking. In that kind of encounter, neither person listens to the other properly. Practice in this activity should help you experience what it's like to listen carefully and attentively, and will stand you in good stead to develop the practice of active listening with your patients and colleagues.

---

3. Interpreting accurately

In interpreting what at first appears to be dubious information voiced by a patient or colleague, it is important to avoid immediately forming a prejudicial opinion on what has been said. Instead, a careful assessment of the extent of the other person's level of understanding may be required. To this end, it is also useful to collect any cues from non-verbal information and assess the extent of this influence on what has been said. To make this estimation, you will use as your baseline your own experience or level of knowledge and expertise about the situation or condition. It is then possible to make a judgement or evaluation on the accuracy of this understanding, which can then be utilised, for example to help a patient gain further understanding of health advice on weight management or to improve accuracy of a procedure in the case of a fellow student. Therefore, interpreting means gathering information before you form a judgement and explanation of a situation or events, with the intention of improving understanding.

Interpreting messages is also a form of translating, and you may be called upon to translate from one language to another. A frequently occurring example of this is changing the bioscientific terms used in medicine into everyday language, to enable understanding or meaningful comprehension on the part of patients. It could also involve taking a complex idea and transforming it into a simpler and more understandable idea that is related to the real-world situation of the patient or setting.

4. Giving clear instructions

This is a skill that requires practice and is harder than it seems. One way to become accomplished is to talk through what you are doing as you are carrying out an activity, and (this is most important) say why you are doing what you are doing.

As a general rule, when working directly with patients, always begin with the simplest explanation and work towards the more complex. This is invaluable when you are carrying out procedures with patients whom you require to participate but who may be anxious. In these situations gradual exposure to information is needed so that their anxiety is not further increased by unnecessary information, and the information should be paced according to their information needs. However, when teaching a skill to colleagues, a different tack is needed whereby all the information will need to be transmitted; yet this can also be in a graded and staged approach to facilitate assimilation and retention of information.

5. Behaving in a professional manner

As a nurse, you have a legal and moral duty to maintain your competency and to work within the scope of your practice. There is an expectation that you will act in a professional manner, and establish realistic boundaries related to time, purpose of the interaction and level of involvement with patients and those in your care. These principles can also relate to interactions with fellow students and nursing and other healthcare colleagues. Intrinsic to these principles are notions of respect for basic human dignity, cultural openness, sensitivity to individuals' circumstances, an understanding of the impact of ill health or disability, and an adherence to standards of care. Conveying these attributes to your colleagues and patients is an important part of demonstrating your professional awareness and competence. A further consideration is the use of research evidence to improve nursing practice, which can be integrated into your educator role through, for example, patient information on health-promoting activities and informational presentations for colleagues.

6. Communicating information clearly

The first step to communicating clear information is to know your audience and what they will accept as a preferred means for messages to be communicated. Questions to consider are: which language is being used (jargon or lay terms), what dialect is needed (nurses need to switch from one form of language to another in relation to dialect or generation), whether humour is acceptable, the extent and limits of confidentiality, whether the messages should be personalised, whether learning styles are an important factor to consider, and whether a different style is required for children, adults with learning difficulties or aggressive patients.

The next step is to decide whether the message is task- or relationship-oriented. An example is the instructions given by flight attendants before take-off. If humour is injected to gain your attention, are you annoyed, as you believe it trivialises the information, or does it make you sit up and listen? The task is the information about safety procedures, whereas the relational aspect is the inclusion of personalised remarks that could either reduce or exacerbate tension. You will have to decide which approach to use by knowing your audience. There will be times when the task is the most important aspect of the communication, perhaps in emergency situations, and there will be other occasions when the more relational aspects will be paramount.

When all these factors are considered, the appropriate message medium can be selected to transmit the information. Selection of message medium now, of course, includes the use of contemporary information technologies as well as written and verbal models of message transmission.

As part of the NHS reforms in 2011, the government set out to consult on how information is communicated via different technologies to patients in *Liberating the NHS: An information revolution* (Department of Health (DH), 2011). It is part of the government's agenda to create a revolution for patients – *putting patients first* – giving people more information and control, and greater choice about their care. In August 2014 the NHS opened up a consultation on the proposal to make sure hospitals, GP practices and other NHS and social care services provide information that meets NHS England's Accessible Information Standard (NHS England, 2014a). More attention is being paid to how information is given to patients and in formats that are understandable and accessible. A more technical approach is from the development called Patient OnLine, an NHS England programme initiated in August 2014 (NHS England, 2014b). This will promote online services to patients, including access to records, online appointment booking and online repeat prescriptions. To support this development is a Patient Working Together Group to ensure a patient-centred approach at every stage of the implementation.

The information revolution is about transforming the way information is accessed, collected, analysed and used by the NHS and adult social care services. Key themes in the consultation are:

- patients having access to and control of records;
- different channels for care delivery, for example, e-mail;
- standards for records;
- outcomes frameworks rather than process targets;
- transparency and openness;
- setting data free for research and other secondary uses;
- information to support better self-care and choice.

We have been concentrating on the communication between nurses and patients, but in the future you will have to consider your role in how technology is used to communicate messages, which may require you to learn new skills with new and developing technologies. This is an opportunity for nurses to take the lead in developing **informatics** skills. On an individual communication level you will need to think about assisting patients in navigating and understanding information resources to enable more self-care via sources such as the internet. For your own development you will need to use information technology resources proactively to keep up to date with current practice, such as telemedicine, telenursing and remote nursing (for a selection of resources on new developments in this field, see useful websites at the end of the chapter). You will be expected to access and use patient clinical diagnostic information to inform clinical decisions and to use information to help deliver more effective care, in order to meet quality standards and audits of clinical care.

Patient satisfaction with healthcare is most often rated more highly when nurses recognise a person's fears and worries. This can be transmitted succinctly with a few words. Similarly, if students feel their personal needs are recognised, they will respond to information receptively. However, if the patient or colleague is sending out signals that s/he only wants to know the task-related information, then this is what is needed.

7. Establishing credibility

As a student, you may believe that you have little credibility as an educator, yet credibility can also equal believability, which is the ability to inspire belief or trust. You may wish to consider how you could demonstrate these characteristics to others in a manner that may not rest solely on your nursing knowledge, but more on the type of person you are or are becoming. In the early stages of your course, you may feel unable to take on the responsibility of teaching others. However, as you progress through the programme, even moving from one year to the next, you will be in a position to help more junior students with advice and information. Credibility is also about your acceptability among your colleagues, and demonstrating that you can be reliable or helpful can generate acceptability. The perception that a person is competent, knowledgeable and skilled enhances credibility. Demonstrating these characteristics in areas where you have proven your ability, such as through examinations or presentations to your colleagues, is particularly effective in strengthening interpersonal relationships.

> ## Case study: Sarah's presentation
>
> *Sarah is coming to the end of her second year and, although anxious about this, wants to consolidate her practice learning experience with a presentation of what she's learnt to her nursing and other healthcare colleagues. She uses Microsoft Office PowerPoint to help make the presentation seem as professional as possible, while balancing this with lively and appropriate images that she's downloaded from the internet.*
>
> *The presentation goes very well and she receives positive feedback about it from all of her colleagues. This gives her confidence to do this more often in the future.*

Communication and health promotion

Earlier in this chapter we proposed that a student has the opportunity to become an educator in many different situations. One that is becoming increasingly important is as an advisor on promoting health and well-being. The World Health Organization (2000b) called for the explicit inclusion and application of health promotion in all nursing curricula. Twelve years later a study by Walthew and Scott (2012) demonstrated that student nurses had difficulty in understanding the concepts of health promotion and health education and that students used information-giving techniques without any notion of empowering individuals to understand their own health needs. The text *Health Promotion and Public Health for Nursing Students* in the Transforming Nursing Practice series (Evans et al., 2014) explains in detail the concepts involved in understanding empowerment and would be a useful reference for further reading.

In a small study of pre-registration nurses, Holt (2008) found that students could learn to look for opportunities to communicate health messages in the healthcare assessment process. The prompt for this learning would be from modules exploring health promotion or public health concepts and theories. Healthcare assessment, however, is often viewed as a tick-box, checklist activity and, with the differentiation of tasks to care assistants, may not be completed by qualified nurses. This does reduce the opportunities for dialogue between an informed practitioner and a patient or client to communicate health promotion or prevention messages. The key is to look for opportunities where health messages can be communicated and to understand how this can be started. You may want to check this out with your mentor first.

Understanding the triggers can only be achieved if you know what to look for, which is why it is important to be knowledgeable about any condition or situation that you are going to discuss with the patient or client first. Know your facts and the current research or related evidence. With so much information available to the public on health matters on the internet or in the media your role may be to sift through the information with patients and guide them on the evidence that is underpinning the information, using your knowledge of critical evaluation of research or evidence.

Evans et al. (2014) suggest that, when talking to people about health matters, you need to think about how you will translate jargon or technical language into language that can be understood, yet not be patronizing. The key in this situation is to find out what the person already knows and what s/he understands. From here you can clarify and explain any unknown terms and provide correct information where there are misunderstandings. This step-by-step approach helps to build a partnership between you and the person. It is also important to divide the information into manageable 'chunks'. Too much information can overload anyone, especially if they are feeling unwell or anxious, and these states of mind can also affect a person's retention of information. If you introduce a stepwise approach to the conversation patients will be able to absorb the information and nurses can facilitate deeper learning (understanding) as opposed to just memorising superficial information (surface learning).

The student as lifelong learner

The NMC *Standards for Pre-registration Nursing Education* (2010) stress that nurses should commit themselves to lifelong learning, and think in a future-directed and nursing field-related way. This idea was first articulated by Basil Yeaxlee and Eduard Lindeman in the 1900s, when education was proposed as a continuing aspect of everyday life (see Falk, 2014). The notion of learning throughout life is not new, as a peep into the Greek philosopher Plato's work, *The Republic*, written nearly two and a half millennia ago, reveals. Initially, lifelong learning was seen as adult learning and was deemed to be for learning's sake and therefore non-vocational. It was seen to build upon existing formal education, to extend beyond formal education providers to groups, such as religious or union groups and societies, and build upon a belief that individuals will see the value of education and will therefore become self-directed learners.

A gradual shift has taken place for lifelong education to be reconceptualised as lifelong learning. The world we inhabit has seen economic, social and cultural change, where many live in a 'knowledge' or 'informational' society, characterised by continual striving to keep up with technological and societal developments. The result is that adults now take part in many non-formal learning activities, such as short courses, study tours, membership of fitness centres and sports clubs, heritage centre activities, self-help therapies, consulting management gurus, electronic networks and self-instructional videos.

The importance of skills

The increasing importance of skills in the UK population is seen as a major challenge when set against world economic forecasts for global economies. This may seem a lofty ambition, and far removed from your studies as a student nurse. Yet, the implications for you and your future working life are that you will need to be aware of the demographic changes that are impacting qualified practitioners in the health field as well as people in all walks of life.

We in the UK are not in a position to be complacent, as the demand for high-level skills is going to increase as global competition for resources also increases. Our population continues to age, and there are rapid changes in technological developments. We are relying more and more on innovation to drive our economic growth. The ability to do this relies on a nation's skills and knowledge. Currently, our nation's skills are not world-class. National productivity trails many of our main international comparators. The UK has high levels of child poverty, poor employment rates for the disadvantaged, regional differences and high income inequality. It is perceived that improving skill levels can reverse these trends.

Your future career path will be guided by many factors, ranging from your personal circumstances to your career goals and aspirations. You may wish to become an advanced or specialist practitioner and these roles are well established in many fields of nursing, such as renal nursing and diabetes, and these nurses often undertaken further studies to expand and consolidate their specialist knowledge. They are often remunerated at Band 6 on the Agenda for Change pay band scales. The role of advanced practitioner is not yet fully embedded in nursing practice or recognised within a regulatory framework, but there are many examples of advanced practitioner roles developing in all fields of nursing practice, particularly in primary care, and these are usually remunerated at Band 7 in the Agenda for Change pay band scales. The Department of Health published a position paper on advanced-level nursing (Department of Health (DH), 2010). It provides a benchmark that is generic in that it applies to all clinical nurses working at an advanced level, regardless of area of practice, setting or client group. It describes a level of practice, not specialty or role, that should be evident as being beyond that of first-level registration. The benchmark is viewed as a minimum threshold. It comprises 28 elements clustered under the following four themes (as agreed by expert practitioners):

- clinical/direct care practice;
- leadership and collaborative practice;
- improving quality and developing practice;
- developing self and others.

Consultant nurse practitioners at Band 8 are fewer in number, but have been established in fields such as intensive care, child protection, older persons' health and mental health.

Even if you decide to stay and are comfortable as a Band 5 staff nurse, there is every likelihood that, due to changes in technology and the moving frontiers of knowledge, you will be required to learn new skills and acquire new knowledge. Indeed, to remain a registered practitioner you will be required to meet the NMC standards for continuing registration by completing 35 hours or five days of learning in the previous three years and 450 hours of practice in each area of registration. Lifelong learning will be integral to your continuing professional knowledge and competence. You may also wish to continue to learn and develop areas of knowledge that give you additional interest and pleasure in life. Alongside this will be your continuing development of CIPS at each stage of your professional life.

Chapter summary

In this chapter, we have looked at three stages of learning opportunities for students. Rather than concentrate on the classical approach to study skills, which can be found in a number of other excellent textbooks such as those listed at the end of this chapter, we have taken a path that discusses how students can integrate theory with practice. There is no doubt that learning for reality should be the goal for nursing students as they combine theory with practice. We have suggested that this can be achieved by experiential learning and have provided a model to develop this skill. The relevance of reflective learning was established, although there remain concerns that learning styles are an important consideration if reflection is to be effective. Guidance on how to achieve a skilled performance has been provided for skills development. The role of the student as educator was explored, and guidance has been given for achieving effective communication in healthcare settings. Finally, the relevance of lifelong learning, both personal and professional, has been examined and we have given brief consideration to future career possibilities following completion of the course.

Further reading

Arnold, E and Boggs, KU (2007) *Interpersonal Relationships: Professional communication skills for nurses*, 5th edn. Philadelphia, PA: WB Saunders.
This is a useful text for teaching health promotion and health education.

Evans, D, Coutsaftiki, D and Fathers, P (2014) *Health Promotion and Public Health for Nursing Students*, 2nd edn. London: Sage Publications.

Howatson-Jones, L (2013) *Reflective Practice in Nursing*, 2nd edn. London: Sage/Learning Matters.
This book is an excellent introduction to reflective practice.

Maslin-Prothero, S (ed.) (2005) *Baillière's Study Skills for Nurses and Midwives*. Oxford: Bailliere Tindall.
This is a useful and practical study skills text.

Useful websites

http://www.businessballs.com/kolblearningstyles.htm
This site has details on Kolb's learning styles inventory, and a brief comparison with Honey and Mumford's variation on the theory.

http://www.campaign-for-learning.org.uk/cfl/yourlearning/whatlearner.asp
This site gives more information about Honey and Mumford's learning-styles inventory, providing an outline of the four styles and suggestions for your preferred learning methods.

Chapter 6
The environmental context of communication and interpersonal skills

Chapter aims

By the end of this chapter, you should be able to:

- understand how different care settings might undermine the practice of safe and effective CIPS;
- describe the importance of physical and social-environmental factors in the practice of good communication in healthcare and be able to identify examples of each, in relation to communication within and between groups, families and populations.
- understand what is meant by the terms **prejudice** and 'schema development' and their relation to language use in nursing;
- appreciate the demands placed on CIPS in British nursing by the nature of multiculturalism;
- identify the ways in which institutional racism impacts on communication and interpersonal exchanges in British nursing practice and the ways in which healthcare organisations defend themselves from accepting that they may be institutionally racist;
- describe the meaning of the 'fallacy of individualism' as it pertains to CIPS practice in British nursing care.

Introduction

The environmental context of CIPS for nurses includes multidisciplinary team practice and interprofessional working, across different care settings, within a safe environment. The *Concise Oxford Dictionary of Current English* (Thompson, 1995) defines 'safety' in two ways, one positive and one negative: first, as free of danger or injury, affording security and being free of harm; and, second, in terms of being cautious, unenterprising and consistently moderate.

The first definition seems both helpful and non-contentious. The second, however, might speak to the use of 'safety in practice' in anti-therapeutic, risk-averse ways, which can undermine the deployment of good CIPS (see the section on pages 116–117 entitled 'A specific environmental example: endless rows of chairs' for illustration of this point). Clearly, different care settings will either promote or undermine the concept of 'safe environments'.

With the above in mind, this chapter will begin by introducing you to a discussion of the importance of CIPS within multidisciplinary team practice and interprofessional working, across different care settings and populations, within safe environments. A specific case study will be presented of sexual abuse within a care home. This case study is intended to help you recognise the relationship between a lack of safety and a breakdown in communication within a specific care environment.

The discussion will then turn to the ways in which physical and social-environmental factors are key to shaping communication, and this will be illustrated with the ways in which the physical environment of nursing care can undermine the possibilities for good communication. With regard to the social environment, communication within and between populations, groups and families, and between young and older people, will be discussed and illustrated with appropriate examples. It will be argued that such communication takes place at conscious and unconscious levels simultaneously and utilises power to the advantage of some groups and the disadvantage of others.

Next, we will help you explore the interrelated concepts of prejudice and schema development. These concepts (introduced in Chapter 2) have emerged from developmental psychology and, together with the role of language use, are extremely important in understanding how CIPS can break down in specific healthcare environmental contexts.

Then we will discuss the impact of shifting friendship, family and cultural networks on communication and interpersonal behaviour and skill development. The demands on CIPS arising from British multicultural society will then be contrasted with institutional racism, and its impact on communication, in healthcare environments.

The chapter will end with a critique of the tendency emerging from humanistic psychology to view CIPS as solely located within the individual. In the light of the preceding argument, this 'fallacy of **individualism**' will be seen both to be naive and to convey an overly optimistic picture of human interaction.

Multidisciplinary team practice and interprofessional working

The demands of two or more professional groups communicating effectively within the same team are considerable. When environmental factors are added to the melting pot, the recipe for danger can increase in an alarming way. The following case study demonstrates a specific example of a phenomenon prevalent in recent years, and makes for disturbing reading.

Case study: Communication and sexual abuse of the elderly

On 25 February 2001, The Guardian *newspaper reported an example of the sexual abuse of an elderly woman in a nursing home. In 1991, she suddenly stopped taking her medication. At that time, her family made the assumption that this behaviour was related to an inevitable progression of her slide towards Alzheimer's that had begun some years earlier. However, soon afterwards, she started to exhibit terror each time her formerly beloved son-in-law entered her room at her nursing home. Again, her family made sense of this in terms of her illness progressing very quickly.*

It was only when the owner of the nursing home was arrested for sexual attacks on the elderly women in his care that the family began to piece together a number of strange incidents that had escaped their notice at the time. By that point the old lady had died. Her daughter was of the opinion that her mother wasn't listed as a victim in the court case because the authorities didn't seem to want to discuss what had happened. She further asserted that none of the people whose mothers were abused in the home knew what was going on.

The owner of the nursing home, a man in his mid-60s, was sentenced to four years in jail. That was in 1997. But it seems a cultural and statistical certainty that the sexual abuse of old people by care workers is still going on today and could be as common as that suffered by children in the days before the paedophile problem was recognised and achieved contemporary significance..

*Some years later, the Director of the website and helpline Action on Elder Abuse (**www.elderabuse.org.uk**) expressed the view that sexual abuse of elderly people in care and nursing homes was extremely prevalent. She stated that the helpline received lots of calls from frantic families and care home staff concerning extreme sexual abuse in these homes, and was of the opinion that the number of calls grossly under-represented the true level of abuse taking place. She gave the view that individuals suffering from mental and physical frailty were perfect victims for such abuse, given that they can't defend themselves or get away from the environment they find themselves in.*

She added that, in her view, such abuse was more about power than sex, and that there were even pages on paedophile websites encouraging men finding it hard to access children to gain employment at care homes.

Catalogue of assault

According to Action on Elder Abuse (2011), there are five main types of abuse in care homes:

- *physical* – including hitting and restraining, or giving too much, or the wrong, medication;
- *psychological* – shouting, swearing, frightening or humiliating a person;
- *financial* – illegal or unauthorised use of a person's property, money, pension book or other valuables;
- *sexual* – forcing a person to take part in any sexual activity without his or her consent;
- *neglect* – depriving a person of food, heat, clothing, comfort or essential medication.

Activity 6.1 — *Team working and research*

As a group doing an internet inquiry, investigate the extent to which any of the above has changed since the early 1990s. You can use the web resources at the end of the chapter to help you.

- What safeguards are in place to protect the vulnerable?

Hint: The aim of this activity is to help you develop your skills in critical internet searching.

The environmental impact on communication

The importance of environmental factors in skilled interpersonal communication was argued in Chapter 3 (Hargie and Dickson, 2004). To recapitulate, Hargie and Dickson argued the crucial relevance of the *person–situation* context for making sense of interpersonal communication. Hendricks and Hendricks (1986) supported this standpoint earlier from the perspective of social-environmental theory, which emphasizes the environment as a very important factor in shaping communication. With regard to the elderly, for example, the residential healthcare environment produces both opportunities and constraints between staff and patients, generally and specifically, around communication. As can be seen from the above worst-case scenario of sexual abuse, communication between staff and patients, and between patients and their relatives, can be seriously compromised under conditions of extreme exploitation of patients.

The exploitative exercise of power in such a circumstance can stay undetected and unreported when staff, and some relatives, engage in selective attention, rationalisation and denial. This might be played out when people choose not to notice certain disturbing facts because it clashes with their own interests. For example, nursing staff in a rest home may not want to recognise signs pointing to the home owner's serial abuse of residents because of a fear that 'going public' about this might result in them losing their jobs, and along the way becoming very unpopular with some of their colleagues. Conversations about the possibility of such abuse then become forbidden territory, although the uncomfortable, non-verbal behaviour of some nurses will be telling.

The physical environment

The 'environment' in this theory is defined as both physical and social. At the level of physical environment, the layout and shape of the building can both provide opportunity for, and constrain, good interpersonal communication. In illustration of this, Nussbaum et al. argue that:

> the architectural design of a nursing home can 'control' the interaction within the building. If the nursing home is designed with a central nursing station and has residential wings extending from the center, it is very unlikely that individuals who are placed in separate wings will enter into a relationship. Proximity is a primary factor for selecting an individual for interaction, and the architecture often dictates who will be close both physically and relationally.
> (Nussbaum et al., 2000, p14)

A specific environmental example: endless rows of chairs

Alec Grant spent some time in the early 1980s as a charge nurse in an acute unit for mentally ill older people. Throughout his nurse training, he had noticed the tendency of chairs on ward dayrooms, especially on wards for older people, to be in a row against the dayroom walls. In his view, also expressed by many other nurse writers and practitioners at the time, this reinforced isolation and prevented communication among patients.

In this author's first few days in charge of the acute unit, he imagined he had the power to make environmental changes to improve communication by changing the position of the chairs in the dayroom to allow for, rather than inhibit, communication among the patients. The chairs were arranged in small circles of four and the intention was to keep them this way and observe for any increase in communication between the patients. When he next came back on shift he noticed, to his dismay and irritation, that the chairs had been moved back to their original position in rows against each wall. Once again, he had them moved back into small circles of four, but each time he went off duty they were moved back against the wall.

This rearrangement of the chairs went on for several days until he found out that the ward cleaners, with the blessing of their managers, had been moving them back to their original positions to ease their cleaning duties. He found his own nursing management unsupportive of his idea of moving chairs to improve communication on 'health and safety' grounds ('the patients might trip over the chairs'). This example of a failed experiment aimed to improve communication between patients clearly illustrates the double-sided nature of safety mentioned in the introduction to this chapter. Questions arise as to who wins and who loses in this picture of chairs placed in rows in the interest of 'safety'.

The social environment

Communication with and within groups, families and populations will vary in style, content and function. Researchers working in the related areas of social identity theory and self-categorisation theory argue that group norms influence behaviour when the social identities with which they are associated are meaningful to the individuals in the group (Hogg and Vaughan, 2011). Put more simply, people in different social groups will experience social identities that 'work' precisely because other members in their particular group experience themselves as having similar or complementary social identities.

Social identities will correspond to specific sets of attitudes, behaviour and communication styles, and, for some people, to **culture** and **ethnicity** (to be discussed more in Chapter 7). Their ability to adapt to their new circumstances is also likely to depend on the flexibility of their personal schemas (see Chapter 2), the strength of their social identity (which might be antagonistic to the new set of people they find themselves in), their mastery of the language used in the new social environment (see discussion on both of these topics below); their age; their perception of how safe they feel; and perhaps numerous other factors. We will now consider these principles and issues in the context of using CIPS with children, adolescents and teenagers.

Communicating with Children
Nina Dunne

Getting the Right Start: The National Service Framework for Children, Young People and Maternity Services – Standards for Hospitals (Department of Health (DH), 2003, p16) states that:

> *For children and young people to participate fully as partners in their care they have to have access to accurate information that is valid, relevant, up-to-date, timely, understandable, developmentally ethically and culturally appropriate. A range of communication methods should be developed and used . . . in a variety of formats, media and languages.*

Children have a right to effective communication in the healthcare setting. Indeed, the United Nations Convention on the Rights of the Child (United Nations, 1989, p4) asserts that *Children have a right to be consulted, to be heard, to express their own views and feelings.* Communication supports everything that children's nurses do. Effective communication skills are therefore crucial in developing professional and therapeutic relationships with children and young people and this is embedded in the theory of family-centred care.

There is also a moral obligation to communicate effectively with children (Department for Children, Schools and Families, 2004; United Nations, 1989) and therefore they need to be treated as active partners in the care that affects them and be allowed to exercise choice and have the right to make decisions (Department of Health (DH), 2003). When children are treated as active partners, adherence to treatment regimes and cooperation with treatment can improve (Tates and Meeuwesen, 2001). Children also appear less upset and recovery rates can improve.

However communication with children is generally neglected (Levetown, 2008) and some healthcare professionals continue to describe children as beings who are not yet able to understand and communicate in an appropriate manner and therefore who are not able to contribute to the therapeutic relationship (Tates and Meeuwesen, 2001; Favretto and Zaltron, 2013). However, it has been found that very young children tend to be more accurate in providing information about their health status than their parents (Riley, 2004). Also excluding children can cause them to experience a sense of abandonment (Clarke et al., 2005). Children's enhanced understanding provides a sense of control of the situation, and their perceptions of their value in the situation are important due to the relationship between their self-esteem and self-worth and medical outcomes (Prilleltensky et al., 2001).

Communication difficulties

When communicating with children, you need to consider their developmental age as well as their chronological age. The environment and situation will also affect the child's level of communication as anxiety and unfamiliarity can cause difficulties with communication. Many children can pick up on body language and facial expressions and misunderstandings can occur if the child perceives a difference between what is said verbally and non-verbal communication. Therefore you need to be aware of gestures and facial expressions as this can hinder communication.

When communicating with a child who has communication difficulties it is helpful to gain the assistance of the parent/s in interpreting what has been said. The use of interpreters and translators can confer both benefits and problems. Professional translators are aware of cultural issues and can diffuse situations where questions that are considered inappropriate for that culture have been asked. Professional translators can be an effective aid in communication. In this kind of scenario, the use of relatives may not be appropriate, however, as this may be an upsetting and stressful situation and confidentiality issues may also arise.

Levetown (2008) has developed three elements for *physician–parent–child communication*:

1. *informativeness*: quantity and quality of health information provided by physician;
2. *interpersonal sensitivity*: affective behaviours that reflect the physician's attention to, and interest in, the parents' and child's feelings and concerns;
3. *partnership building*: the extent to which the physician invites the parents (and child) to state their concerns, perspectives and suggestions.

In extrapolating from this to nursing practice, it is important that informativeness matches the cognitive needs of the child and family and therefore you must be able to assess the developmental level of the child in order to communicate effectively. This forms the basis of healthcare professional *task-related behaviour* (Levetown, 2008, p1442).

Interpersonal sensitivity and partnership building address the affective needs of the patient and/ or parent, thus focusing on their emotional needs. It is important that the child and family feel heard and not just talked at. Feeling heard constitutes *relational behaviour* (Levetown, 2008, p1442) and partnership building is central to family-centred care and shared decision making.

Communicating with children of different ages

Teaching children how to communicate with the healthcare professional has been found to be effective (Lewis et al., 1991). This work suggested that children taught in this way preferred an active role in their care and felt they had a better experience whilst in hospital as a consequence.

Infants: Birth to 12 months

In order to develop language skills, infants need exposure to speech and therefore it is essential that nurses talk to infants and toddlers and interact with them in order to stimulate them. Infants also need to be able to see the face of the person speaking to them and, as distance sight is still developing, it is important that the nurse is close to the infant to maintain eye contact.

The tone of voice is also very important and infants respond to a voice with both a higher pitch and a sing-song quality. Infants tend to communicate through coos, gurgles and grunts, although facial expressions and more extensive body language are also used. It is important that the nurse is able to get the help of the parent when trying to interpret these sounds and movements. When you carry out interventions with children in this age band, it is important that you talk through and describe procedures as you are doing them.

Toddlers: 12 to 36 months

Toddlers communicate with a combination of gestures, grunts, one-word sentences, two-word sentences, positive and negative emotional expressions and body movements. They can assign meanings to words. They do want to be able to express themselves, so patience on the part of the nurse is required. Parental involvement to help in interpretation may also be useful. The implications emerging from this for you is that, in the context of separation anxiety, you may be seen as a stranger so trust needs to be established first. Discussion and explanation of a procedure should occur immediately before its implementation.

Pre-schoolers: 3 to 6 years

Pre-schoolers begin to talk in full sentences that are grammatically correct. Young pre-schoolers may struggle with accounts in the correct order, but by age 6, sequencing the events comes much more easily. However, they can still easily misinterpret conversations and have a short attention span. In this regard, it is important that you explain the procedure that is about to be carried out with reference to all the senses: that is, what the child will see, smell, taste, hear and feel, and that you are honest about the pain that the child may feel.

School-age: 6 to 12 years

School-age children talk in full sentences, much like adults. They ask more questions, can relate past experiences in vivid detail and seek more information and justification for the way things are. Moreover, school-age children can handle receiving more pieces of information at the same time compared with pre-school children. All of this points to nurses using books and pictures to explain procedures. Children within this age band are developmentally ready to handle detailed explanations. However, it is important that you do not patronise the child; ask children how much information they would like.

Some communication techniques

In attentive listening, the nurse pays attention to verbal and non-verbal cues and is attempting to understand the content and the feelings behind the discussion. However, making assumptions about what the parent or child wants to say, judging the parent or child and allowing the conversation to get off track can be barriers to attentive listening.

Using silence can encourage parents to speak by giving them time to think through the information and consider the alternatives. However, silences should not be allowed to go on too long as this can become uncomfortable.

The use of questioning can help with clarification. Open questions allow the parents to respond in the way that they choose and can encourage disclosure, but the conversation can get off track. So questions should be focused and not too general. Closed questions can make the parents feel that they are being rushed and, although useful for clarifying information, they can be leading.

Communicating with parents

Children's nurses need to communicate with parents as well as the child. Poor communication with parents can affect their recall and therefore adherence to treatment regimes (Hallström and Runneson, 2001). It has been found that parents need information that is timely even if it is distressing (Perrin et al., 2000). Some parents also want advice which can put the nurse in a difficult situation. Above all, parents want to feel that they are being listened to. Parents also want to be involved in how their children are informed (Tates and Meeuwesen, 2001) and the amount of information their child is given. However, it is important that nurses are mindful that this may conflict with the needs of the child and can hinder his or her treatment and recovery because, as already mentioned, enhanced understanding can provide the child with a sense of control.

Activity 6.2   *Communication*

As a group, work on the following scenario:

Three-year-old Alice has difficulty breathing and is showing signs of respiratory distress. She has laboured breathing and is obviously uncomfortable. Alice's observations are within normal limits; however her respiratory rate is 24 respiratory rate per minute. Her hands and feet are cool and pale. Alice's mother is quite tearful and emotional seeing her child like this. Alice's father is angry that nothing is being done quickly enough to help Alice and is questioning everything that you are doing.

- What is the goal of communication with the patient and parents?
- What are the challenges of communicating with the patient and parents in this situation?
- Would communication without the parents present help the situation?
- How will you achieve this?

Hint: This exercise will help you think through some of the complexities of working with children in this kind of healthcare scenario.

Communicating with adolescents and teenagers

Chris Cocking

As a qualified nurse you will routinely come into contact with adolescents and teenagers – young people – in clinical practice, whether or not you choose to work specifically in paediatric nursing. It is therefore vital that you are able to communicate effectively with them.

Activity 6.3   *Team working and reflection*

In a group, before reading further, explore your attitudes towards teenagers and adolescents (you might be one yourself). Identify the ways in which perspectives expressed are related to the ages of people in the group.

Twelve- to 18-year-olds are often categorised into a unified social group ('adolescents' or 'teenagers') that is feared and/or pathologised in society and popular culture, amusingly illustrated in the collection of clips on YouTube of the comedian Harry Enfield's character, Kevin. However, because it is a stage that everyone goes through on their path to adulthood, it is important that you build on your understanding of the physical and psychological challenges experienced and how this may influence individual communication styles and development. First of all, it's worth highlighting that not all scholars see this period of transition as an objectively fixed concept and Thurlow (2005) suggests that the concept of adolescence is more of a social and economic construct than determined solely by age or biological changes. Furthermore, young people's categorisation as a single homogeneous group (e.g. 'teenagers') is often imposed upon them by adults. For instance, Williams and Garrett (2005) argue that young people may come to identify as a group at least in part because they are often uniformly treated as such a group by adults and their associations with their peers are often demonised and/or curtailed.

However, while young people's associations with each other and the resulting peer pressures they can experience are often considered as negative influences and responsible for a variety of negative outcomes (including involvement in gangs, and the development of eating disorders), their social networks can also be a source of support and strength that help them deal with the challenges of adolescence (Drury, 2015). There is evidence (Fortman, 2003) that young people rate communication with adults less positively than with their peers, and that this dissatisfaction is at least in part due to the perception that adults fail to engage effectively with young people, which could explain why young people may be reluctant to communicate with adults. Fortman suggested that viewing adolescent communication and behaviour from an intergroup perspective would be more beneficial than merely looking at individual communication styles. Furthermore, in a review of adolescent communication with adults in authority, Drury (2003) argued that antagonistic representations of how adults view communication skills in young people (and vice versa) could contribute to a vicious cycle of poor mutual interactions, with adults considering that young people have poor motivational and communication skills, and young people highlighting the power imbalance and lack of respect that adults have for them as contributing to the communication difficulties they experience. However, merely framing the issue in terms of helping young people to improve their communication skills could also deflect responsibility from adults looking at possible deficits in their own communication, and so Drury (2003) concluded that any efforts to 'improve' young people's communication skills need to be considered in a broader context of unequal group relations.

Challenges in communicating with young people

The issue of communication has clear relevance for how young people engage with health professionals, and so it is vital for nurses and other health workers to consider how they engage with such a client group. Poor communication could not only reduce the effectiveness of health interventions if young people do not follow advice from professionals, but could also result in them avoiding engagement with health services altogether if they feel their needs are not being considered or understood. Wrate (1992) found that doctors perceived adolescent patients as sullen or even hostile, and it seems likely that this could in turn affect how they then interacted with them, however good they believed their own interpersonal skills were.

A common cliché is that young people can be uncommunicative (any parents of teenagers may well be used to grunts, one-word answers, shrugging of shoulders and the term *whatever* when their offspring talk to them!). However, the reasons for such communication difficulties are more complex than teenagers simply losing the ability to speak in words of more than one syllable. For instance, Drury et al. (1998) found that when young people reported communication difficulties with parents, this was because of a lack of a shared point of view or unwillingness to hurt the parents' feelings. When looking at communication difficulties with their employers, lacking the courage to speak out was listed as a more common reason.

Therefore, if faced with an uncommunicative young person in hospital, rather than putting it down to typical teenage behaviour, it is worth trying to find out any possible underlying reasons for this unwillingness to communicate and seeing if you can help improve the situation. For instance, a young person admitted to accident and emergency may be scared, disoriented, in pain, or even unwilling to be there (especially if s/he has been brought in by an anxious parent). So, recognising the distress the young person may be in, and helping to devise strategies to deal with such fear and uncertainty could help improve effective communication. Giving the young person space to communicate without the parents present can also be useful if any parent–child dynamics are escalating the situation (although be aware that this can often require equally good communication skills with the parent when requesting privacy to communicate with the young person!).

Young people's use of language can be a source of mystery to adults and they often use phrases and/ or slang that may appear strange, or sometimes inappropriate and grossly offensive. One contentious example of this is that, although the term 'gay' is often used by teenagers in a disparaging way to describe others, it arguably may not be intended as a form of homophobic abuse. Clearly, while it can still be perceived as offensive by those hearing the term, a survey in 2008 found that 83 per cent of teachers heard pupils use the term in insults, but also reported that its use was almost never related to sexual orientation or activity (**http://news.bbc.co.uk/1/hi/7289390.stm**). Although this survey may be read as simply illustrating how offensive language may be used relatively innocently, such a reading is in line with and reinforces the heteronormative assumption that using the word 'gay' in this context is harmless because the young people who do so *are not really being homophobic*. The fact that 83 per cent of teachers maintained that the use of the word in this context was not homophobic needs to be balanced with the fact that many young gay people will become distressed when they overhear these kinds of conversations. Further, how might the teachers have responded if they had heard the word 'black' used instead of 'gay'? Would they have explained this away so innocently?

Irrespective of how this survey is interpreted, the boundaries of appropriate language still clearly need to be enforced. That said, nurses may need to separate out what may be socialised usage of language by young people without fully understanding its possible implications and what constitutes a concerted attempt to oppress others through the expression of prejudiced attitudes, and respond appropriately in both instances. The reasons for young people creating their own communication styles (and sometimes their own language) can be varied, but Fortman (2003) argued that young people often define themselves through how they verbally interact with others. This can be a strategy to maintain a positive sense of group identity that is different from adults, which is in line with Tajfel's (1982) social identity and Turner et al.'s (1987) self-categorisation theories from social psychology that suggest people seek positive self-esteem by categorising themselves into social groups with similar others with whom they identify.

Therefore, a word of caution is necessary before you run off to learn the latest guide to teenage slang. Although it's good for nurses to understand and be able to engage with young people, it's also important to realise that they may resist adults using 'teenager language'. This is because part of the reason for its use is to gain positive in-group distinctiveness by communicating in a way that sets them apart from adults, as predicted by Tajfel (1982), and this process can be undermined by adults trying to reappropriate their terms.

Cultural awareness

Since the majority of communication is non-verbal, there is more to communicating with young people than being familiar with the language they may use. Therefore, it is vital to be aware of ways that young people may communicate with others by culturally expressing themselves. There are currently a variety of youth subcultures in the UK (such as Goths, Emos, Metallers, Ravers, Skaters), and each has its own style of clothes and behavioural norms that may influence how they interact and communicate with adults. Nursing staff need to be accepting of these different forms of cultural expression, and engage with the young person in a non-judgemental or discriminatory way, however bizarre or even offensive they may find the young person's dress sense or bodily piercings.

These subcultures can sometimes be linked to reasons why young people come into contact with health services, but this should not be allowed to influence your interactions negatively. For instance, Young et al. (2006) found that identifying with Goth subculture was strongly associated with deliberate self-harm and suicide attempts amongst young people in central Scotland, so nurses may need to be sensitive and non-judgemental when dealing with such clients who may present with evidence of deliberate self-harm.

If you find that you share some social or cultural interests with your clients, this may be a way of initially engaging with young people and can help encourage trust and the creation of a therapeutic relationship. However, you also need to be clear about the need to maintain effective professional boundaries, so that you can present an appropriate role model to sometimes impressionable and/ or vulnerable clients, and that you don't find yourself in awkward situations with your clients or other colleagues. For instance, younger qualified staff and/or student nurses who find it easier to identify with the young people they work with could be perceived as being a softer touch than older/more senior staff, and so more susceptible to attempts at manipulation by clients.

Case study: A hypothetical scenario

Consider the case of Vicky, a 22-year-old newly qualified nurse who identifies as being from the Goth subculture. She has just been offered a job working with young people aged from 12 to 18 in an inpatient unit. She passed the interview with flying colours, but was told by the local manager that she needs to present herself as an appropriate role model when working with vulnerable clients, and this means that when working on shift, she should dress appropriately and remove any facial piercings for her own safety. She also used to self-harm by cutting when she was 15 or 16 to help cope with a depressive episode she experienced after being bullied at school and has long scars down her arms (although she hasn't self-harmed since). It has been agreed that she can disclose her own experiences of self-harm if she thinks it will be helpful for her to develop a sense of empathy with particular clients who are otherwise difficult to engage with, and/or as a therapeutic tool to show that it is possible to come through such episodes and develop other forms of coping. However, she has been advised that she needs to exercise good judgement in this matter, and be aware of the need to maintain appropriate professional boundaries. Therefore, it has been agreed that she will cover the scars on her arms when working on the ward and/or in groups, but is allowed to reveal them during one-to-one sessions with clients if she considers it appropriate.

Think about the benefits of following this approach and any possible challenges that Vicky might experience from clients and/or other colleagues.

Communicating via technology

It is worth discussing the technology young people use to communicate with each other and how it may affect nursing practice. The last 15 years have seen an explosion in young people's use of IT devices and social media (mobile phones, tablets, iPads) (Coleman, 2011), and parents could be forgiven for thinking that their teenage children are unable to survive without being in constant contact with their peers via the latest device that is in vogue. Nursing practice needs to keep up with such advances in communication technology, and most clinical environments now have policies on the use of mobile phones while in hospital (NHS, 2009). In some Child and Adolescent Mental Health Service inpatient environments, young people may be allowed to keep their mobiles with them while admitted, as they could be a useful way to keep in contact with the outside world to reduce feelings of isolation and/or homesickness while in hospital. However, staff may also reserve the right to regulate their use if they have any concerns regarding possible safeguarding issues arising from their use. For instance, young people often swap numbers with each other on admission in an effort to make friends within the new social group, and unfortunately peer dynamics sometimes mean that people fall out with each other and bullying by text could happen when adolescent friendships break down.

Disclosure

As a nurse, you will often be interacting with young people when they are removed from their natural environment, and this can involve confusion and fear for them. However, this can also be an opportunity for you to converse with them when they are less susceptible to the social norms of 'teenage' behaviour, meaning that there is sometimes space for them to open up in a way that they may not feel they can do with their parents, teachers or other significant adults in their lives. This can result in young people disclosing information to you about themselves or others at risk, and so you have to be clear that you have a statutory duty to pass on any information about possible safeguarding issues. This can place you in a position of both great trust and responsibility, and so it is important that you do not make promises you may not be able to keep if a client asks you not to pass on information s/he has disclosed to you (especially if s/he is under 16, or has other capacity issues).

Concluding comments

Communicating with teenagers and adolescents can feel like a thankless task at times, with adults fearing they can say nothing right. However, it need not be such a source of mystery and/or trepidation, and can even be rewarding at times. An ability to empathise with their needs and concerns is vital, as well as to take time to consider the perspective they may have in your interactions with them. Finally, it always helps to have a good sense of humour and never hurts not to take yourself too seriously when working with them.

Competing narratives informing social identity

Mindful of how group and individual identities are formed according to social identity and self-categorisation theories, it is worth considering related ways in which interpersonal communication within the clinical nursing environment may be influenced by implicit differences within and between some nursing and client cultures, around what is taken for granted but not usually openly expressed. On the basis of narrative research, Grant et al. (2014) discuss how mental health staff and clients in their study storied the same events in mutually antagonistic ways on the basis of different narratives informing the motivations and experiences of the two groups. These authors argue that institutional mental health staff tend to privilege their storied explanations of events and the clients in their care as *the truth*, thus marginalising and dismissing the ways in which clients make sense of their, often distressing and abusive, experiences. This trend of 'culture-centrism' is played out in relationships between younger nurses and older people.

Communication between younger nurses and older persons

Some key issues of interpersonal communication between nurses and patients on the basis of group differences will be discussed later in this chapter. For the moment, consider the ways in which differences in speech and language, and overall communication, between, for example, young and older people, can often be marked. Younger nurses may assume that the way that they speak and dress is right and proper, and needs no justification, without considering the impact of all of this on people in their care. Although they may consider that they are providing a good standard of care, they may equally fail to notice how their dress and conversational style exclude and disrespect patients. In this regard, as also stated in Chapter 7, the social-environmental communication context for nursing practice is crucial, and ethical and professional violations can easily occur because of the unquestioned dress and behaviour code of some employees.

Another stark example of nurses not paying sufficient attention to the person–situation context is in the use of what has been described as 'baby talk'. Ryan and Hamilton (1994) studied nurse–patient interactions with elderly nursing home residents. Some nurses demonstrated a lack of respect in their use of baby talk, and related voice tone and parental style. Nurses and volunteers using baby talk were rated less respectful and competent than their peers and elderly recipients of such baby talk were, clearly understandably, less satisfied with the interaction.

The use of baby talk and inappropriate clothing and styles of talking raises interesting questions about how many healthcare workers, including nurses, take for granted the cultural assumptions they have about themselves and the world and others within it, and, in related terms, their power relative to others. These questions alert us to the need to be mindful of how such assumptions develop, and also how they may be seriously compromised in the face of demands made on nurses working sensitively with groups and populations who are gaining the confidence to challenge the constraints imposed on them by normative assumptions. The contemporary social emergence of trans communities highlights this issue.

Prejudice and schema development

From a cognitive developmental perspective, none of us are born with psychological maps or templates for understanding the world, other people or ourselves. These develop over time, mostly in childhood, as a result of our interactions in the world with significant others, particularly our parent or parents. Described as schemas, or core beliefs (Grant et al., 2008, 2010), they are necessary to equip us to make sense of ourselves in interactions with others and in changing life circumstances and situations.

Those of us fortunate enough to have good enough parenting will develop schemas (see Chapter 2) which enable us to get by relatively reasonably successfully in the world, and with other people and ourselves. However, equally, because of abusive early life experiences, many of us will grow up with a core sense of ourselves as 'worthless', 'bad', 'useless' or something equally self-denigrating, which can lead to troubled relationships and sense of self throughout life.

Research and practice summary: Schemas as 'self-prejudice'

In her ground-breaking work on helping the kind of people described immediately above, Padesky (1991) explains how she helps her psychotherapy clients begin to consider how their deeply held negative schemas are a form of 'self-prejudice'. She does this by asking clients to bring to mind someone in their life who is deeply prejudiced. This prejudice may, for example, be directed towards certain groups of people because of their religious or sexual orientation. She then engages in a dialogue with them to help them review the ways in which such prejudices may be maintained through forms of selective information processing. This can include attending to information that confirms the 'truth' of the prejudice, while ignoring or discounting evidence that challenges it. Clients are then invited to consider the similarities between their own deeply held negative schemas and the prejudices and prejudiced people they have been discussing.

Activity 6.4   *Evidence-based practice and research*

Log on to **www.padesky.com**. From there, follow the links to 'Clinical Corner' and left-click on 'Pubs'. In this page you will find Padesky's article 'Schema as prejudice'. Read this article and discuss it in small groups in your class. Consider possible implications for interpersonal communication in your work as a nurse.

Hint: This activity should help you understand better not only that all of us develop psychological templates for understanding ourselves, the world and others, but also that sometimes such templates can be deeply prejudicial.

A strikingly ironic feature of deeply held prejudices, whether – in Padesky's terms – they are prejudices held against oneself or directed towards societal groups, is that they are often not experienced or regarded by the people who hold them as prejudices at all. Instead, they are considered to be right and proper, and common sense – a reflection of the world as it is, rather than a distortion of reality or a bigoted point of view. In order for people to begin to rid themselves of their prejudices, they would have to begin to question them and see them as contingent (dependent on events and circumstances in their upbringing) rather than as absolutely true.

Nursing and dominant cultural beliefs

It may be helpful at this stage to consider the extent to which we all hold such culture-centric beliefs and assumptions about our life-worlds that remain taken for granted as 'just so' rather than potentially or actually problematic. Parfitt (1998) suggests that the majority of nursing care is delivered from the value position of nurses, and that this may therefore be based on their dominant cultural beliefs.

Narayanasamy and White argue that:

> *Ironically, the vast majority of indigenous healthcare workers have rarely, if ever, previously given consideration as to what their values and cultural beliefs are. Or how their values, beliefs and cultural traditions are acquired. Yet most assume, with equal measures of ignorance and arrogance, that their 'British' culture is the right way and that it is naturally superior to all other 'uncivilised or unsophisticated' cultures. Regrettably, those who possess that chauvinistic attitude will come into conflict with patients/clients who are not Anglicized or 'British'. That negative tension or cultural conflict, if not rapidly dispelled, will ultimately undermine the therapeutic relationship between patient and [nurse]; and therefore the quality of care will be compromised.*
> (Narayanasamy and White, 2005, p104)

Padesky, and other cognitive psychotherapy writers (Hayes and Smith, 2005; Grant et al., 2008, 2010) argue that prejudices and other forms of deeply held belief are maintained through engaging in speech and language, and related behaviour, that give form and substance to the prejudice.

In this regard, there are two interesting views of the world that may be useful to contemplate: in the first, the world is more or less separate from the language we use to describe it; in the second, the world is constituted or given shape, substance and reality by language.

Theory summary: The Sapir–Whorf hypothesis

That language defines the way a person behaves and thinks was argued by Edward Sapir (1983) and his student and colleague Benjamin Whorf (1956). Both believed that language and the thoughts that we have are somehow interwoven, and that all people are equally affected by the confines of their language. In short, they argued that all people are, in a sense, mental prisoners, unable to think freely because of the restrictions of their vocabularies.

An example of this idea is apparent in George Orwell's famous book *1984*, in which he discusses the use of a language he calls 'Newspeak', which was developed to change the way people thought about the government. The new vocabulary they were given was created to control their minds. Since they could not think of things not included in the vocabulary, they were, by default, zombies, imprisoned by the limits of their language. Sapir and Whorf coined the term *linguistic determinism* to capture the notion of ideas and creativity as the prisoners of vocabulary. If people indeed cannot think outside the confines of their language, the result of this process is many different world-views by speakers of different languages.

According to Sapir and Whorf, an idea complementary to linguistic determinism is 'linguistic relativity', which states that the differences in languages reflect the different views of people from different cultures. A key question emerging from this perspective is that if the world-view and behaviour of people are shaped by the structure of their language, and languages differ across cultures, then what are the threats to coherent cross-cultural communication and understanding in the modern world?

The Sapir–Whorf hypothesis would indicate that absolute conceptual barrier-free communication seems unlikely. There is no question that the vocabulary of a specific language emphasises particular things, objects, events and experiences in a culture. For example, a society where horses are revered will have many words for horses and horse-related things because people in this society will talk about their horses a lot. Similarly, the Inuit people have many words for snow, the North Americans for cars and the Norwegians for fish. Now this does not necessarily mean that people from other cultures are incapable of perceiving the items that are described with such specific vocabulary, elsewhere. However, they are likely to nuance the meanings of these items through the perceptual lens related to their own specific cultures.

(Continued)

(Continued)

In criticism of the Sapir–Whorf hypothesis, if the English language was somehow keeping us from freedom of thought, we would all be trapped in the same cognitive path if we were English speakers. However, people from different cultural and ethnic backgrounds speak English as their main language, and even among siblings and close relatives, the understanding of certain words and what they mean varies. This is due to different environmental shaping factors to which people in the same family have been exposed, or expose themselves; to personal interests, friends and teachers, and perhaps to age and generation differences. If we were totally prisoners of our language, two people living in the same house with the same genetic make-up and speaking the same language should think and talk identically about issues, things, people and events. This is obviously not the case. That said, awareness of, and discussion around, the contribution of the Sapir–Whorf hypothesis are important components of globalisation, communication and cultural education in the world today.

If the Sapir–Whorf hypothesis is accepted as useful to a greater or lesser extent, the degree to which we are all more or less 'trapped within' language in making sense of, and constructing, our worlds has fairly clear implications for nursing people from different cultures – and this includes cultures of ethnicity, race, sexuality, religion. For example, something that one cultural group takes for granted, in relation to healthcare and communication, may be alien and experienced as deeply strange by another group. This is made all the more complex by the fact that, within one culture, there may be many shifting, constantly evolving and changing subcultures. Wikipedia defines a 'subculture' as a group of people with a set of behaviours and beliefs that could be distinct or hidden, and that differentiate them from the larger culture to which they belong. This means that, as nurses, we must be very cautious about making rash cultural assumptions. It is easy, for example, to interact with people on the basis of a cultural stereotype which we think such people may immediately relate to and connect with, but which may be experienced as presumptious and offensive by them.

Shifting friendship, family and cultural networks

It was argued above (Hogg and Vaughan, 2011), on the basis of social identity theory and self-categorisation theory, that social identity is experienced in relation to the primary reference group to which a person belongs, be it family and/or friends or colleagues. Within the space of a lifetime, an individual is likely to shift primary reference groups several, perhaps many, times and develop identities and related values and communication styles different from, and possibly in opposition to, their original reference groups.

Such shifts may appear radical in form. For example, the 1960s saw the emergence of Flower Power and Psychedelia. A decade later, the Punk and Anarcho Punk movements emerged, partly in reaction against the music, style, attitudes and forms of communication associated with Psychedelia, followed more recently by, among others, the Grunge and Goth movements. Such youth- , music- and style-related movements have been described as 'subcultures'. Subcultures exist in opposition, or run counter, to the dominant cultures within which they are embedded, while employing elements, materials and motifs from those cultures in novel ways to generate new cultural meanings (Hebdidge, 1979).

Within Britain, in addition to sub- and **countercultures**, shifting populations with their different health needs – for example, refugees – are currently moving within and between changing social contexts such as family structures and friendship networks. With regard to ethnic differences alone, this gives rise to a rich and complex multicultural picture, which has clear implications for the need for skilled interpersonal communication, and related awareness, among nurses.

Institutional racism

Insensitive behaviour to people from different ethnic groups, whether it results from deeply held prejudices, ignorance or simply thoughtlessness, can often produce organisational pictures of institutional racism.

Case study: Institutional racism

The Macpherson Report (1999) suggested that most of Britain's public institutions displayed institutional racism, defined as:

The collective failure of an organisation to provide an appropriate and professional service to people because of their colour, culture or ethnic origin. It can be seen or detected in processes, attitudes and behaviour which amount to discrimination through unwitting prejudice, ignorance, thoughtlessness and racist stereotyping which disadvantage minority ethnic people. *(Macpherson of Cluny, 1999, p10)*

Case study: Rocky Bennett, Roger Sylvester and Sean Rigg

Google 'Rocky Bennett Inquiry' and read the websites that come up. In October 1998, David 'Rocky' Bennett died as a result of forced restraint by up to five nurses at the Norvic Clinic psychiatric inpatient unit. Preceding this event, he was the victim of sustained institutional racism by both staff and clients alike. Narayanasamy and White (2005) assert the belief that institutional racism pervades healthcare, including nursing. It certainly seems to be the case that Rocky Bennett was the tragic victim of this problem, but how representative of a more general trend is this? One thing is certain: ask many nurses if it goes on in their workplace and they'll deny it. This kind of response represents a kind of defensive 'NIMBYism' ('not in my back yard') that should alert the enquirer to the possible operation of organisational defence mechanisms (Morgan, 2006).

You may also want to compare the material from the Rocky Bennett websites with two more recent examples of the death of black men in the mental health and police systems:

(Continued)

(Continued)

Roger Sylvester died in 1999 after being restrained by six police officers in a mental health unit in Haringey: **http://en.wikipedia.org/wiki/Death_of_Roger_Sylvester**

Sean Rigg, who had mental health problems, died in police custody in Brixton in 2008: **http://en.wikipedia.org/wiki/Death_of_Sean_Rigg**

Developing the propositions of psychoanalyst Sigmund Freud, Morgan (2006) argued that organisations, in terms of their collective worker mindset, are just like individuals in using unconscious protective measures to escape blame. Table 6.1 illustrates this argument in relation to institutional racism and related interpersonal communication difficulties.

According to Morgan (2006), organisational defence mechanisms, by definition, occur at an organisationally unconscious level. In relation to this, healthcare organisations have a tendency to socialise many of their members into a 'silent and tacit' agreement with the organisation's values and 'the way things are done around here'. Because of this, nurses may relatively rapidly forget the idealism they had when training in favour of buying into the kinds of organisational communication styles and difficulties described above.

The fallacy of individualism

A difficult but necessary question to pose is to what extent mainstream approaches to the dissemination of CIPS in nursing are culture-centric – embedded in cultural values. A criticism of the widespread reliance on counselling models of interpersonal communication to inform interpersonal skills books in nursing has already been discussed in this book. Developing this argument from the position of **culture-centrism**, it can be argued that Rogerian (see pages 43–45) and related humanistic influences in CIPS in nursing betray the assumption of a taken-for-granted individualism.

From an individualistic standpoint, patients and nurses are assumed to have the innate psychological ability to find their own solutions to their problems, independent of the cultural, organisational, social or material constraining factors which both give rise to such problems in the first place and maintain them. Individualised solutions include being able to speak more effectively and genuinely through communication facilitated by therapy and counselling workers employing the Rogerian core conditions. This assumption, which has a long legacy in the psychological therapies, has been contested vigorously from a critical psychological position (Smail, 2011), challenging the overly simplistic idea that people can somehow rise above or effectively combat these constraining factors solely by their own efforts (see, for example, Grant and Leigh-Phippard, 2014).

Related to these critiques of individualism is the fact that environmental, organisational and cultural discourses (world-views) both shape and limit what can be done and said in any interpersonal exchange among nurses, between nurses and other healthcare workers, and between nurses and patients. Complementing the Sapir–Whorf hypothesis, discourse theory argues that

Defence mechanism	Defence mechanism defined	Possible communication difficulties
Repression	Pushing unacceptable ideas and impulses into the unconscious	The possibility that abuse and communication neglect go on in our organisation is relegated to the organisational unconscious
Denial	Refusing to acknowledge a disturbing fact, feeling or memory	Presenting a public face of transculturalism while maintaining institutionally racist forms of communication and refusing to acknowledge this at an organisational level
Displacement	Shifting disturbing feelings aroused by one person on to a safer target	Maintaining that 'it is not our responsibility to display culturally sensitive forms of communication because we have not been trained in it'
Rationalisation	The creation of elaborate or unconvincing schemes of justification to disguise underlying motives and intentions	'Racism does not go on in our organisation. Difficulties in communication between nurses and ethnic minority patient groups are due to circumstances outside our control, including the failure of those patient groups to adapt sufficiently to take advantage of the care on offer'
Regression	Adopting behavioural patterns found satisfying and effective in childhood in order to reduce the effect of uncomfortable demands	Sending ethnic clients 'to Coventry', by avoiding them and avoiding talking with them
Splitting and idealisation	Inappropriately separating different elements of experience, and talking up the good aspects of a situation to avoid facing the bad ones	'We represent a centre of excellence in many aspects of our care and this has been acknowledged by feedback from many patients and articles in the local press'

Table 6.1: Organisational defence mechanisms (adapted from Grant et al., 2004)

none of us can avoid speaking from a particular discursive position (Speed, 2011). To put this more simply, there is no vocabulary or set of actions available to us, to talk about, and relate to, our worlds – professional and otherwise – which are free from cultural meaning shaping that has already taken place before our entry into those worlds.

In spite of the above difficulties with the individualistic stance, deriving from selective aspects of humanistic psychology generally (Whitton, 2003) and Rogerian counselling more specifically (Rogers, 2002), a simple, naive and overly optimistic picture of human interaction emerges. This is about two or more individuals interacting in a cultural and organisational-environmental vacuum.

The humanistic picture of interaction in Figure 6.1 both contrasts with and masks a more challenging image of the nurse and patient interacting within multiple cultural and organisational environmental contexts, which have the power to shape and limit what can be said and done in the name of 'communication and interpersonal skills in nursing' (Figure 6.2).

Figure 6.1: Simple picture of interaction

The individualist/counselling model of skilled communication

There is no such thing as society.
(Margaret Thatcher, 1987)

By placing sole responsibility for good CIPS on nurses, the organisation is let 'off the hook' for the kinds of environmental factors, described above, that work to undermine good communication (Grant, 2002). At a local cultural level, the kinds of unwritten rules, also described above, resulting from socialisation into organisations, impact on communication styles (Morgan, 2006). These rules, often held at an unconscious level, will affect the quantity and quality of communication between different professional groups and between health workers, including nurses, and patients.

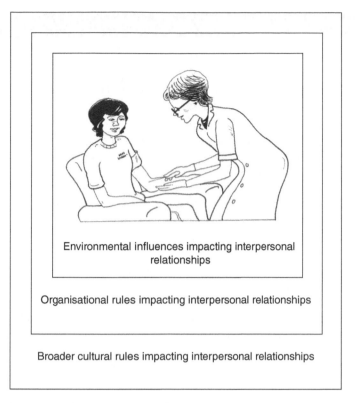

Environmental influences impacting interpersonal relationships

Organisational rules impacting interpersonal relationships

Broader cultural rules impacting interpersonal relationships

Figure 6.2: Complex picture of interaction

Task, rather than holistic patient, workplace cultures will result in 'I–it' rather than 'I–thou' relationships (Buber, 1958). At a broader cultural level, institutional racism and sexism, and cultural incompetence, and the prejudice that accompanies these problems, are often likely to influence the quality and quantity of nurse–patient interpersonal communication, but, unfortunately, remain under-acknowledged or denied.

Chapter summary

Different care settings may undermine the practice of safe and effective CIPS. Physical and social-environmental factors are very important with regard to the practice of good communication in healthcare, in relation to communication both between and within groups, families and populations, and between younger and older people. 'Prejudice' and 'schema development', and their relation to language use, are key to understanding examples of poor CIPS in nursing. Institutional racism impacts negatively on communication and interpersonal exchanges in British nursing practice.

There is a variety of ways in which healthcare organisations defend themselves from accepting that they may be institutionally racist. The 'fallacy of individualism' in CIPS practice in British nursing care masks the important role of environmental, organisational and broader cultural influences impacting upon such care.

Further reading

McDougall, T (2006) *Child and Adolescent Mental Health Nursing.* Oxford: Blackwell.

Rutter, M, Bishop, D, Pine, D, Scott, S, Stevenson, J, Taylor, E and Thapar, A (eds) (2010) *Rutter's Child and Adolesecent Psychiatry,* 5th edn. Oxford: Wiley-Blackwell.
Useful reading for working with children and adolescents.

Cioffi, J (2006) Culturally diverse patient–nurse interactions on acute care wards. *International Journal of Nursing Practice,* 12(6): 319–325.

Leininger, M (1997) Transcultural nursing research to nursing education and practice: 40 years. *Image Journal of Nursing Scholarship,* 29(4): 341–347.
One hundred culture-specific studies by Madeleine Leininger.

Nussbaum, JF, Pecchioni, LL, Robinson, JD and Thompson, TL (2000) *Communication and Aging,* 2nd edn. Mahwah, NJ: Lawrence Erlbaum Associates.

As the titles of the above references suggest, engagement with them will help you become more familiar with research on transcultural nursing practices and on communication both between and with elderly clients.

Useful websites

www.bjmp.org/content/uncovering-face-racism-workplace
This is an interesting 2009 article on racism in healthcare and other work settings.

www.elderabuse.org.uk
This is a national resource on the issue of abuse of the elderly in care and nursing homes.

www.socresonline.org.uk/15/3/8.html
This is a sociological article focusing on conceptualisation of institutional racism and related policy following the Rocky Bennett inquiry.

Chapter 7
Population and diversity contexts of communication and interpersonal skills

NMC Standards for Pre-registration Nursing Education

This chapter will address the following competencies:

Domain 2: Communication and interpersonal skills

1. All nurses must build partnerships and therapeutic relationships through safe, effective and non-discriminatory communication. They must take account of individual differences, capabilities and needs.

3. All nurses must use the full range of communication methods, including verbal, non-verbal and written, to acquire, interpret and record their knowledge and understanding of people's needs. They must be aware of their own values and beliefs and the impact this may have on their communication with others. They must take account of the many different ways in which people communicate and how these may be influenced by ill health, disability and other factors, and be able to recognise and respond effectively when a person finds it hard to communicate.

NMC Essential Skills Clusters

This chapter will address the following ESCs:

Cluster: Care, compassion and communication

4. People can trust a newly qualified nurse to engage with them and their family or carers within their cultural environments in an acceptant and anti-discriminatory manner free from harassment and exploitation.

By the first progression point:

1. Demonstrates an understanding of how culture, religion, spiritual beliefs, gender and sexuality can impact on illness and disability.
2. Respects people's rights.
3. Adopts a principled approach to care underpinned by *The Code* (NMC, 2008).

Introduction

Society today is enriched by multicultural, ethnic and social, sexual, gender and religious diversity. The focus of this chapter will be on the interpersonal and ethical contexts of nursing people from such different backgrounds and cultures. By looking at how populations have evolved in the UK, we will begin by studying the statistical data on **immigration** and **migration** to help understand how diverse ethnic populations in many of our neighbourhoods have developed. We will also explore the motivators behind human migration.

The chapter then divides into two sections, with one focusing on cultures and the next on diversity. Beginning with cultures, we will take into account the range we experience in nursing and the differences that make up a society of diverse groups and identities. Culture is a sociological concept and we will be investigating some of this terrain to gain a deeper understanding of the diversity (the differences between people) and the potential for discrimination. We will concentrate on communicating in the context of cultural diversity by exploring concepts such as cultural preservation, negotiation and repatterning, or restructuring. These are interventions that are geared to changing previously held patterns of behaviour that can have a major detrimental effect on patients' lives and are linked to discriminatory practices.

We explore some of the issues of nursing in a multicultural Britain and the need for cultural awareness and cultural competence, and we compare two theories of **transcultural** care.

The chapter goes on to examine diversity and socio-economic position, as well as taking time to explore and understand diversity in a society that is made up of different groups, to which power, influence and opportunities are not always equally granted. This section briefly discusses race and culture, gender issues, sexual orientation, age and disability.

We will conclude with a section that considers the ethical and moral consequences of communication and personal interactions.

Populations and diversity

From the earliest of times, the islands that make up the UK have been settled or invaded by many different peoples: Romans, Saxons, Goths, Vikings and Normans. In more recent times, we have seen, as a result of the two world wars in the last century and the harmonisation policies of the European Union (EU) in this century, people from Europe finding sanctuary, work and education in the UK.

Activity 7.1   *Reflection*

Using a range of different sources (e.g. local and national newspapers, magazines, television serials or 'soaps'), make a simple analysis of their portrayal and coverage of peoples of different gender, age, ethnicity or religion. Reflect on any differences between local and national media representations.

- How are messages communicated about culture and diversity in these media?
- Are there any specific references to culture and diversity and healthcare, and how do they relate to your experiences so far in practice settings?

Hint: This exercise should help you gain a better insight into how the media communicate culture and diversity and how this is linked to healthcare.

The UK has a history of colonialism – a policy of acquiring land for exploitation and trade that broadened the economic reaches of the UK and set up administrative systems in many countries around the globe. This in turn established a network of trade, migration and immigration opportunities that led to the UK recruiting colonial subjects in the Second World War as soldiers; it also recruited men from the Caribbean to work in munitions factories and in Scottish forests. After the war, the UK continued to recruit from the West Indies and Commonwealth countries to meet labour shortages in transport and in the NHS. Links with Africa, Asia and the Far East have also developed immigration routes to the UK and people have settled, bringing with them their cultural practices, traditions, customs, religious beliefs and attitudes, thus providing a rich multicultural tapestry. The expansion of the EU in 2004 opened the doors to people from countries such as Poland, the Czech Republic and Slovenia, bringing yet more cultural variety to the UK. Further expansion of the EU member states from 2020 could enable this diversity to expand.

Motivation for migrating

Adventurous nomadic groups and individuals, conquering armies and traders of every kind have migrated across the globe for centuries to seek new opportunities, employment and ways of thinking. Consequently, almost all nation states – not only the UK – are the product of multiple, overlapping generations of immigrants. It is helpful to understand the motivation behind people's reasons for migrating and these can be classified into different categories.

- *Settlers* are people who intend to live permanently in a new country, mostly in the main countries of settlement such as the USA, Canada, Australia and New Zealand. To be a settler you need to qualify in some way: being a skills immigrant, or already having family in the country, are usually the main criteria.

- *Contract workers* are admitted to other countries on the understanding that they will stay only a short time. Many are seasonal workers in the agricultural industry. Included in this category are nurses from the Philippines and Eire who are contracted to work in the NHS for short periods. It also includes students attending university. In nursing, this currently only refers to post-qualifying studies, as the NMC states that only UK citizens can qualify for NMC-regulated pre-registration courses conducted in the UK.

- *Professionals* are people who are employees of transnational companies and who are moved from one country to another. All industrial countries have a system of work permits that regulates the time and scale of residency.

- *Undocumented workers* is a polite term for illegal immigrants. Some have been smuggled into the country and others may have stayed beyond the ends of their work permit.

- *Refugees and asylum seekers* – a refugee is defined by the United Nations as someone who has a well-founded fear of persecution for reasons of race, religion, nationality, membership of a particular social group or political opinion. During the 1990s, more and more receiving governments started referring to such people as 'asylum seekers' and only termed them 'refugees' when their claims were accepted.

These categories are not exhaustive and do overlap. For example, an Indian medical practitioner working in an NHS hospital may be both a professional and a contract worker.

Data on immigration, emigration and migration

A census surveying all people and households in the country is undertaken every ten years in England and Wales, the most recent one being undertaken in March 2011. This census provides essential information from national to neighbourhood levels for government, business and the community. Data are also collected on immigration, emigration and migration, and collated by the Office for National Statistics (ONS) through the Annual Population Survey (APS). Being informed with accurate data on the reasons why populations migrate and the extent of migration into the UK not only helps nurses to understand the reason why people move from one country to another, but also reduces the myths and prejudices that sometimes lie behind beliefs held about immigrants and asylum seekers. The web resources at the end of the chapter give you the links to the most current data. The data presented here are current at the time of going to press. Estimates of the population by country of birth and nationality from the June 2010 APS (Economic and Social Data Service (ESDS), 2010) show that 88.6 per cent of the UK population were UK-born and 92.8 per cent were British nationals (Table 7.1). British nationals are people who have British citizenship, either because they were born with it or have been granted it since. Nationality is not necessarily determined by country of birth. This compares with estimates of 88.7 per cent of UK-born and 92.9 per cent of British nationals in the year to June 2009.

In the year to June 2010, a total of 40.7 per cent of UK residents not born in the UK had British nationality. Of those UK residents who did not have British nationality, 5.8 per cent had been born in the UK. In the year to June 2010, India was the most common country of birth for UK residents born outside the UK, and Polish was the most common non-British nationality (Table 7.2).

	British national (%)	Non-British national (%)	Total (%)
UK-born	88.2	0.4	88.6
Non-UK-born	4.6	6.8	11.4
Total	92.8	7.2	100.0

Table 7.1: UK residents by nationality and country of birth: estimates for year to June 2010 (from Economic and Social Data Service (ESDS), 2010)

Non-UK country of birth	Estimate in thousands	Non-British country of nationality	Estimate in thousands
India	678	Poland	541
Poland	520	Republic of Ireland	342
Pakistan	421	India	322
Republic of Ireland	398	Pakistan	165
Germany	292	USA	150

Table 7.2: UK residents by non-UK country of birth and by non-British country of nationality: estimates for year to June 2010, top five (from Economic and Social Data Service (ESDS)P, 2010)

The main reasons for migration to the UK are for work or study purposes. Different nationalities have different visa requirements for entering and staying in the UK, for example, European Economic Area and Swiss nationals do not require a visa to come to the UK. For over 100 other nationalities, covering three-quarters of the world population, a visa is required for entry to the UK for any purpose or for any length of stay. For all remaining nationalities a visa is required for those wanting to come to the UK for over six months, or for work.

Excluding visitor and transit visas, most entry clearance visas are issued under the points-based system for work (Tiers 1, 2 and 5) and study (Tier 4). Entry clearance visas also include those for family reasons. The total number of entry clearance visas for work and study issued in the year to December 2010 was 501,475, similar to the levels in the year to December 2009 (503,540). Of the entry clearance visas issued in the year to December 2010, a total of 166,660 were work-related. This was an increase of 3 per cent on 162,450 in 2009.

The available data (see the web resources at the end of the chapter) start at the year to December 2005. The highest number of entry clearance visas issued for work-related reasons into the UK was 260,640 in the year to December 2006. This figure declined gradually to 158,975 in the year to March 2010 and has since remained at a similar level. The number of entry clearance visas issued for the purposes of study, including Tier 4 (students) and student visitors, was 334,815, a decrease of 2 per cent on 341,090 in 2009. In the year to December 2005, a total of 210,080 visas were issued for the purposes of study. This figure increased gradually at first, reaching 267,880 in the year to June 2009, but then it increased sharply, peaking at 362,080 in the year to June 2010, a rise of 35 per cent on a year earlier.

Net migration (the difference between immigration and emigration) increased to 198,000 in 2009 compared with 163,000 in the previous year. This change was primarily as a result of decreased emigration. The number of people leaving the UK for 12 months or more fell to 368,000 in 2009 compared with 427,000 in 2008. The drop in total emigration was due to a decrease in the numbers of British and EU citizens leaving the UK. An estimated 140,000 British citizens emigrated in 2009, the lowest number since 1999 and down from 173,000 in 2008. An estimated 567,000 people arrived to live in the UK in 2009, which is consistent with levels seen since 2004 and compares with 590,000 in 2008. Non-British citizens accounted for 83 per cent of all immigrants; a third of these were from EU countries. Immigration for formal study was the most common reason stated for arrival into the UK in 2009, with an estimated 211,000 (37 per cent) compared with work-related reasons (34 per cent). Immigration to the UK for work-related reasons dropped to 193,000 (from 220,000 in 2008) and is at the lowest point since before inclusion of the eight EU accession countries in 2004.

The UK population continues to age gradually. The number of people aged 85 and over reached 1.4 million in mid-2009, comprising 439,000 men and 930,000 women and accounting for 2.2 per cent of the total population. Between 1981 and 2009, this age group increased by just under 0.8 million. The proportion of people aged 85 and over rose from 1 per cent of the population in 1984 to 2 per cent in 2009. It is projected that, by 2034, it could rise to around 5 per cent of the population. While the UK has an ageing population, it is not ageing as rapidly as that of some other countries, such as Germany, Italy and Japan.

Although life expectancy in the UK is improving in line with most western European countries, relatively high levels of fertility ensure that the proportion of the population that is young remains high. There were 11.5 million people aged under 16 in mid-2009 compared with 12 million people of state pensionable age, each age group accounting for 19 per cent of the total population. In mid-2009, there were more people of state pensionable age (men aged 65 and above and women aged 60 and above) than there were under-16s, a pattern first seen in mid-2007. Around one in ten residents of the UK are foreign-born, a lower proportion than in many developed countries. UK population density has increased steadily and is the fourth highest in the EU.

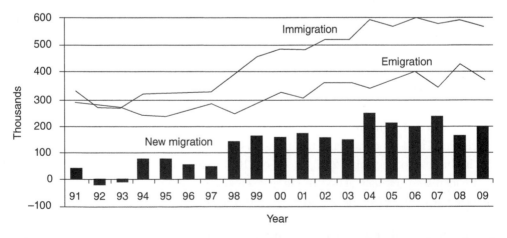

Figure 7.1: Migration (adapted from data from the Office for National Statistics licensed under the Open Government Licence v.1.0)

The gender difference in the population aged 85 and over has decreased over recent decades; in 2009 men accounted for 32 per cent of the population aged 85 and over, and in 1981 they accounted for 23 per cent. In comparison, men accounted for approximately 49 per cent of the total population (all ages) in 2009 and this percentage has changed very little over time. The age and gender structures of the UK population have significant consequences for the health and social care support given to individuals in the future, and will also have an effect on the level of cultural awareness required in communication skills. This is discussed later in the chapter.

Being sensitive to differences

There is a danger that being different from the majority in any society will be equated with being inferior. Thompson (2001) points out that being sensitive to differences prevents:

- *alienating people* by making groups feel that they do not belong in society;
- *invalidating people*, which creates the feeling that views are not valid because they are different;
- *missing key issues* by not noticing crucial factors because we are not sensitive to the significance they have for others;
- *becoming part of the problem*, which is failing to challenge discrimination and oppression and thereby playing a part in their continuance.

Focusing on culture

Culture is a complex and multifaceted social phenomenon that affects our lives. To be an effective communicator with culturally diverse patients, a nurse has to be able to understand different social structures and norms that influence values and behaviour in different societies. By having this knowledge, nurses can understand unfamiliar behaviour patterns and attitudes without dismissing or devaluing them. On a practical level, this requires speaking to patients in appropriate ways with knowledge of culturally congruent language, in order to manage intercultural health-care episodes.

Definitions relating to culture

Let us look at some common definitions. Leininger defines culture as *a common collectivity of beliefs, values, shared understandings and patterns of behaviour of a designated group of people* (Leininger, 1997, p175). The term 'culture' is often used to describe a very large social group based on a shared national origin.

It can also refer to a regional culture reflecting a collective sense of being through activities, traditions and language contained within a geographical area, or to an organisational culture that implies an ethical ethos or political stance.

Generally speaking, culture is a learned social experience that is often handed down through generations, thus providing a continuing connectedness with others in a community. Over periods of time, social rules and norms are established that provide a code of behaviour for the community and that also provide safety and security. Within the culture, there may be differential status roles and yet individuals connected within the culture are regarded as like-minded persons, whereas someone who is not part of the culture can be treated with mistrust and suspicion.

According to Henley and Schott (1999), culture affects every aspect of daily life: how we think, feel and behave, and make decisions and judgements. Culture can be defined as 'how we do and view things in our group', which in large part is acquired unconsciously in early childhood (Hofstede, 1991).

Activity 7.2   Reflection

- To appreciate how culture is learned, identify and describe one family custom or tradition in your own family or community group. Ask your parent, grandparent or an elder where the custom originated. Has the custom or tradition changed over the years and can your relative or elder tell you why?
- Can you also think of a custom that you have adopted, but that is relatively new in your family or social group? Can you trace why this has happened, and the source of this custom?

Hint: This activity might help you understand how some cultures become assimilated into the mainstream, or not, and relates to the following topics of multiculturalism and acculturation.

Multiculturalism is the term used to describe a heterogeneous society in which many diverse cultural groups coexist. All groups will share some general characteristics, while some characteristics will be unique to particular groups within the larger multicultural whole. Bearing in mind the discussion above on migration, which indicates a society that is progressively more mobile, society is increasingly considered to be global due to changes in demographics, the internet and an interdependent world economy. The movement towards shared cultural characteristics and social mores is due to increased interracial marriage or relationships between communities and the increased use of media and the internet to share cultural behaviours and beliefs. Conversely, this can also create a cultural conservatism, where groups invest energy to retain cultural differences in an attempt to ward off change and a diminishing of their cultural beliefs.

'Acculturation' represents an adaptive cultural process whereby biological, environmental and traditional forms of culture adapt to prevailing contextual mores. This enables people to survive and thrive, maintain their economic and social status, and constantly develop and celebrate diverse variations of the traditional forms of their original cultures. This can be seen in groups who have moved from an agricultural life to an urban existence, and is particularly evident in the creation of food and eating rituals, for example TV cooking programmes that teach Asian women how to make club sandwiches. A further example is family size – in many cultures a large family represents security and survival, whereas for survival in an economic and materially dependent industrial society, small families are more prevalent.

'Cultural diversity' describes the differences among cultural groups. Diversity is becoming the norm in our societies rather than the exception and covers a wide range of attributes such as nationality, ethnic origin, gender, sexuality, educational background, geographic location, economic status, language, politics and religion. There can also be diversity within the same societal groups, such as age and work cultures. For example, given the very recent legislation relating to an increase in higher education tuition fees, many of today's 18-year-olds will have a different outlook on the benefits of a university education from their older sisters and brothers.

There is also a cultural diversity in health and social care settings among professions, for example physicians, social workers, healthcare assistants, nurses, administrators, porters and physiotherapists each can have their own cultural identities, rituals and practices that can affect decisions and the allocation of tasks.

Case study: The mental health specialist

Alexandra comes from a mental health nursing background, has a Master's degree in cognitive behavioural psychotherapy (CBP) and is accredited as a CBP psychotherapist, supervisor and teacher with the British Association of Behavioural and Cognitive Psychotherapies. Since coming into post, she has occasionally received requests from a mental health day hospital in her area to provide therapy for clients. When these requests were first made, she found that the system of referral was mostly too informal for her liking, to the extent that day hospital clients often had no idea that they were being referred and why they needed to be in the first place. Moreover, she soon discovered that the day hospital nursing staff making the requests had a poor knowledge of the relationship between psychological disorders and appropriate interventions. On one occasion, this resulted in a client being referred for 'exposure therapy' because of an apparent phobic avoidance of getting on buses near his home. On assessment of this client, Alexandra found that his problem with using these buses was not because of phobic anxiety. It was because a group of local thugs, out to get him because of a vendetta against his family, frequently used these buses.

Alexandra identified cultural differences between the generic mental health nursing service and herself around the communication involved in good 'referral etiquette' (Grant, 2010d), and knowledge of psychopathology and evidence-based psychotherapy. She resolved to address these through a series of teaching workshops for day hospital staff.

Cultural relativism refers to the understanding that cultures are not inferior or superior to one another and that there is no method of measuring the value of one culture against another. Furthermore, within cultures individuals will not only ascribe different levels of meaning and importance to cultural beliefs and behaviours, but will violate them in myriad ways. This means that an individual who appears to belong to a culture may not follow all the practices of that culture, particularly if s/he has adopted elements of acculturalisation. The implications for nurses are that some may have made major modifications in their cultural beliefs to make them either more extensive or more moderate. Consequently, customs, attitudes, rituals and beliefs have to be understood according to the individual needs and standpoint of each patient.

The antonym to cultural relativism is **ethnocentrism**, in which a group believes their nation, culture or group to be superior. There are several examples of this in history; for example Hitler and the Nazis, and more recently, opposing sides in the Balkans. To be proud of one's ethnicity is acceptable, but if this is taken to extremes, cultural oppression is the outcome.

Discrimination is another form of ethnocentrism where groups in society are marginalised, such as the physically or learning disabled, people engaged with mental health services, those in poverty or homeless, and persons with HIV. When access to healthcare is inhibited or age and racial discrimination are at play, these are subtle forms of **ethnocentricity**.

Ethnicity derives from the Greek word *ethnos*, meaning 'people'. An ethnic group is a social grouping of people who share a common racial, geographical, religious or historical culture. Ethnicity is different from culture in that it represents a symbolic awareness of elements that bind people together in a social context. Ethnicity is a deliberate and chosen awareness of norms and symbols, whereas culture does not always involve a conscious awareness and commitment to a cultural identity.

Communicating with cultural diversity

Communication is often the first barrier when considering cultural diversity. The language barrier may be the most obvious difficulty to overcome, and if English is a second language there may not be complete mastery of the terminology and ways of describing problems and symptoms. In addition, there may be conflicting assumptions and expectations about health and healthcare due to culturally based health beliefs. This is, however, the tip of the iceberg, as there are many other, not always evident, cultural barriers that lie beneath the surface. Communication requires recognition of care alternatives, confidence in cross-cultural communication skills and the ability to analyse situations in specifically situated contexts. Leininger (1978) has suggested that there are three possible modes of support: *cultural preservation, cultural negotiation* and *cultural repatterning.*

Cultural preservation

This facilitates the retention or incorporation of helpful or harmless health- and illness-related practices, such as traditional herbal teas and ethnic foods, which are integral cultural practices. Wearing garments that are specific to a designation or talismans that maintain cultural beliefs should be retained, for the meaning and symbolism of these artefacts are important to maintaining health in many cultures. Respect for these artefacts is paramount and they should be valued as inclusive contributions to health maintenance.

Cultural negotiation, or accommodation

This means bringing together the biomedical and the cultural by negotiation and understanding. For example, in some cultures a bed facing in a certain direction can mean the person is facing death, so turning the bed around or finding another bed facing in a different direction can allay fears and improve cooperation. In another example, a family of a terminally ill child would not return the child to the unit on time for his medications. The hospital staff interpreted this as the family refusing treatment and were reluctant for the child to go on outings. On discussion, it was discovered that the family wanted to spend as much time as possible with the child because they knew he was going to die, whereas the goal of the staff was to prolong his life as much as possible by using the therapies they had devised. Negotiation between the staff and the family and exploring the conflicting goals enabled both sides to find a new understanding and a way forward, so that the staff supported the outings and the family made efforts to bring the child back on time.

Cultural repatterning, or restructuring

These are interventions that are geared to changing previously held patterns of behaviour that are having a major detrimental effect on the patient's life. In cases where there are legal consequences associated with beliefs, such as in the case of withholding permission for procedures (for example, blood transfusions, surgery or rights to die), the legal aspects of the situation have to be thoroughly considered in addition to the patient's wishes. For situations of abuse or neglect, referral should be made to specialist services for consultation and actions.

Leininger (1978) has suggested using a template of information for culturally diverse clients, which could be considered as a guide for exploring individual patients' cultural needs and includes the following:

1. *Patterns or lifestyles of an individual or group.*

2. *Specific cultural values, norms, and experiences of a patient or group regarding the health and caring behaviours of their culture.*

3. *Cultural taboos or myths.*

4. *The world-view and ethnocentric tendencies of an individual (or group).*

5. *General features the patient (or group) perceives as different from, or similar to, other cultures in or near their environment.*

6. *The health and life-care rituals and rites of passage to maintain health and avoid illness.*

7. *Folk and professional health–illness systems.*

8. *Detailed caring behaviours and nursing care for self and others.*

9. *Indicators of cultural changes and acculturation processes influencing health care.*
(Leininger, 1978, pp88–89)

The skills that a nurse uses to communicate with patients cross-culturally are an extension of the skills previously discussed in this book. However, they can be embellished by the following suggested questions.

- Can you tell me something about the reasons you are seeking healthcare?

- Can you tell me something about how a person in your culture would be cared for if they had a similar condition?

- Have you been treated for a similar problem in the past? (If the patient answers yes, more information about the precise nature of treatment is elicited.)

- Can you tell me what people do in your culture/community to remain healthy?

- Can you tell me something about the foods you like and how they are prepared?

- Are there any special cultural beliefs about your illness that might help me give you better care?

Multicultural Britain

Britain is regarded as one of the most ethnically diverse countries in Europe (Narayanasamy and White, 2005). Therefore, healthcare providers must deliver a service that is culturally sensitive, competent and appropriate to meet specific and diverse needs (Narayanasamy, 2002). However, Narayanasamy and White (2005) argue from a historical perspective (Cortis, 1993; Wilkins, 1993) that, since its inception, the NHS can be viewed as a service that was created to meet the healthcare needs of the British people. Its provision:

evolved around British social and family patterns, embracing religious and cultural beliefs . . . It responded predominantly to the expectations and health needs of the indigenous population in 1948.
(Narayanasamy and White, 2005, p103)

Theory summary: Ethnocentrism

The process of socialisation into the occupation of nursing carries with it the need to internalise the dominant cultural values. Because of this, nursing is not culture-free, but is embedded in cultural values that pervade all aspects of care, practice and knowledge, including CIPS. So nursing is culturally determined. If this is neither acknowledged nor understood, nurses can be charged with being guilty of gross ethnocentrism (Stokes, 1991). In the words of Parfitt:

Nurses who hold ethnocentric views will be unable to interpret their patients' behaviour appropriately as they will judge it according to the norms of their own behaviour.
(Parfitt, 1998, p52)

The extent to which ethnocentric cultural values still prevail in the NHS is a crucial question. Parfitt sees the NHS as *reflecting the cultural norm of not only the white majority but the middle class white majority* (Parfitt, 1998, p50). From this critical position, privileged white British values and assumptions are taken as 'common sense' and 'right and proper', against which ethnic and cultural minorities are located and labelled as 'the other'. This has obvious implications for the prevalence of institutional racism and witting or unwitting prejudice among healthcare workers.

Sawley (2001) highlights racist incidents in nursing and healthcare. These include black colleagues being referred to in derogatory terms; white relatives being allowed to use the patients' toilets while Asian relatives are barred; white staff making racist remarks against Asians; and Asian patients not being permitted to have large numbers of visitors, while white patients were not subjected to such controls. These practices are clearly reflective of racist prejudice in the wider societal context, which Figure 7.2 may help illustrate.

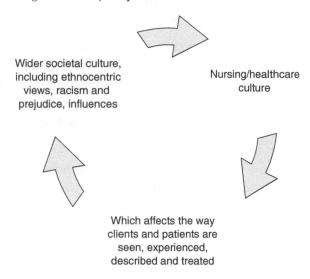

Figure 7.2: Racist prejudice in the wider societal context.

Cultural competence

Cultural competence refers to an ability to interact effectively with people of different cultures. It is comprised of four components:

- awareness of one's own cultural world-view;
- attitude towards cultural differences;
- knowledge of different cultural practices and world-views;
- cross-cultural skills.

Developing cultural competence results in an ability to understand, communicate with, and effectively interact with people across cultures – in short, to be culturally sensitive.

Anderson et al. (2007) explored the principles of involving the community to strengthen cultural competence in nurse education, practice and research in order to reduce the health disparities in communities. The findings of these researchers included the importance of reducing and levelling differences in power between practitioners and the community. It also clearly emerged that communication and relationships between healthcare workers and community members have to be culturally appropriate, and that it was crucially important to work hard to develop trust. Overall, reflecting the importance of the 'I–thou' rather than the 'I–it' relationship discussed in Chapters 1 and 6, it was considered essential that interventions were done 'with' rather than 'to' people.

In a complementary argument, focusing on the experience of pain, Lovering (2006) asserted that patients and health professionals bring their own cultural attitudes to interpret and talk about patients' pain experience, with the health professionals' knowledge and attitudes dominating.

Lovering suggested that this situation could be improved through learning about the differing cultural attitudes towards pain held by both cultural groups and health staff. The rationale for this was that, through such learning, staff and patients from differing cultural groups can work with each other as opposed to the former 'doing to' the latter.

Cioffi (2006) conducted qualitative research in Australia. This explored experiences of interaction between nurses and minority ethnic patients. Nurses and patients from Asian or Middle Eastern Islamic backgrounds were interviewed individually about perceptions of the care provided. Issues identified were tensions arising from the Islamic groups' fear of discrimination, the requirements of visiting relatives, nurses' gender, perceived cultural differences and problems of communication and information exchange.

In support of all of the above, Gerrish et al. (1996) recommended ways in which transcultural healthcare might be transmitted. According to these authors, the overarching need is the development of cultural sensitivity: in this context, the practitioner should assume the role of tourist (with the good manners that go with that role), reflexive honesty (including the ways in which power may be distributed in favour of the health practitioner), exploration of the cultural meanings of ethnicity, striving for intercultural communication and a strong focus to eradicate all forms of racism, including institutional.

Culture without cultural awareness

In the context of ethnocentricity, culture and institutional racism, as with prejudice, the irony is that members of dominant cultures are likely to remain unaware that they have a specific culture. In terms of their social identity, as discussed above, what they regard as normal and universal assumptions, beliefs and behaviours are only 'normal' relative to their class, time and social groupings. In contrast, those who have grown up as minority ethnic group members, or who have lived outside or away from their own society, are much more likely to be acutely aware of the influence of culture by being cultural 'outsiders'.

Transcultural nursing

As discussed in Chapter 1, 'caring' needs to be appraised through a transcultural lens (Leininger, 1997). In related terms, the quest for 'self-awareness' needs to be broadened to subjecting oneself to challenges to one's assumptions (Gerrish et al., 1996), because without the opportunities for self-awareness development in this transcultural sense, healthcare workers are likely to remain insensitive to other cultural values. This speaks to relational ethics (see Chapter 1) in that the imposition of one's own values on others can be offensive and unprofessional (MacNaught, 1994; Baxter, 2000).

In the early 1970s, the second author trained as a student mental health nurse. He witnessed several examples of cultural insensitivity through British nurses renaming their ethnically different colleagues with British names. So, for example, a male colleague from the Republic of the Philippines, whose first name was difficult to pronounce by British colleagues, became 'Fred'. Less understandably, a Danish nurse named 'Elsa' was renamed 'Elsie'.

Fortunately, cultural sensitivity seems to be beginning to impact nursing more now. For example, Narayanasamy and White (2005) argue that healthcare services should be culturally responsive and that the cultural healthcare needs of ethnic minority groups are still not adequately met. Specifically, there is a failure of multicultural education, structures and policies, and transcultural healthcare practice (Gerrish et al., 1996), which may be being met, at least in part, by developing models of transcultural nursing.

The ACCESS model of transcultural nursing

Narayanasamy (2002) offers the following model of transcultural nursing.

- *Assessment*: The assessment process focuses on the cultural dimensions of the client's lifestyle, and beliefs and practices about health.
- *Communication*: The nurse strives for awareness of, and differences in, variations in verbal and non-verbal responses.
- *Cultural negotiation and compromise*: The nurse strives to become aware of aspects of other people's cultures and to understand their viewpoints, and tries to explain their problems in an acceptable and accessible way.
- *Establishing respect and rapport*: What is required is a therapeutic relationship that embodies genuine respect for varieties in culture, beliefs and values.
- *Sensitivity*: Nurses deliver diverse culturally sensitive care to diverse cultural groups.
- *Safety*: Patients are enabled to derive a sense of cultural safety (see the introduction to Chapter 6).

Transcultural care

Robb and Douglas (2004) also addressed social identities – memberships of particular groups said to share common experiences and needs. These are characterised by ethnicity, gender, disability, age and sexuality, all of which structure people's everyday experiences, including being in receipt of healthcare. These can be used to define people as 'other' or 'different', against a supposed 'norm'.

Activity 7.3   *Critical thinking*

A Bangladeshi woman is admitted to hospital for two weeks to undergo an operation. Afterwards, she reports that, while in hospital, she felt stupid because of her lack of English. 'Two nurses neglected me. I'm not sure if it was because of the colour of my skin or because of a language barrier. I'm still not sure what operation I had, and why.'

In small groups, discuss the following questions.

- What is the nature of the communication problem experienced by the woman?
- Whose problem is it?
- What are the consequences for the speaker?

Hint: This activity should help you rehearse some of the transcultural nursing issues you may encounter as a student nurse and post-qualifying.

The questions raised in Activity 7.3 should demonstrate the complexities of the issues, rather than easy answers. The answers you came up with will relate to your understanding of the nature of 'difference', how it is produced and how it should be responded to. For example, one possible answer is that the 'cause' of the problem was the woman's poor command of spoken English coupled with her lack of confidence, either because of her language difficulties or her cultural background.

However, equally, it could be argued that the communication problem arose because of the hospital's failure to address indirect and direct discrimination in its practices. Indirect discrimination was apparent in the failure to take account of the diverse needs of patients by, for example, failing to ensure the provision of bilingual workers or interpreters available for the main community languages in the area. Direct discrimination was apparent in how the two nurses ignored the woman.

The point is that nurses, like all humans, understand 'difference' differently. Related to social cognition-based discussions in this book on labelling, 'cognitive miserliness' (see Chapter 3, page 61) and prejudices, health workers often associate 'difference' with the membership of particular groups. These groups are seen to have specific qualities, ways of communicating and communication needs.

Focusing on diversity

Diversity is about us as individual beings. As discussed earlier, society is made up of a variety of groups and we will explore some of those groups in this section from a sociological perspective. Again, it is these differences that will influence the character and nature of our interpersonal interactions with patients and fellow workers. We will examine socio-economic position, race and culture, gender, sexual orientation, age and disability.

Socio-economic position

This is also described as a person's class and is closely linked to factors such as income, wealth and social status. The ONS uses a classification system to gather data on the population that is constructed around employment roles and economic output. The first detailed classification was designed in 1928 and was intended to identify differences in economic distribution and status.

Social class based on occupation

I   Professional, etc. occupations
II   Managerial and technical occupations
III Skilled occupations

    (N) non-manual
    (M) manual

IV   Partly skilled occupations
V   Unskilled occupations

The occupation groups included in each of these categories were selected in such a way as to bring together, as far as possible, people with similar levels of occupational skill. In general, each occupation group was assigned as a whole to one or other social class and no account was taken of differences between individuals in the same occupation group, for example differences in education. However, for persons having the employment status of foreman or manager, the following additional rules applied:

(a)   each occupation was given a basic social class;
(b)   persons of foreman status whose basic social class was IV or V were allocated to social class III;
(c)   persons of manager status were allocated to social class II, with certain exceptions.

(Adapted from Rose and Pevalin, 2005, p5)

This ethos has prevailed and a further more comprehensive classification system was developed in 1951.

Socio-economic groups

Rose and Pevalin (2005) state that classification by socio-economic group was introduced in 1951 and extensively amended in 1961. The classification aimed to bring together people with jobs of similar social and economic status. The allocation of occupied persons to socio-economic group was determined by considering their employment status and occupation (and industry, though for practical purposes no direct reference was made since it was possible in Great Britain to use classification by occupation as a means of distinguishing effectively those engaged in agriculture).

Classification by socio-economic group

1.1 Employers in industry, commerce, etc. (large establishments)
1.2 Managers in central and local government, industry, commerce, etc. (large establishments)
2.1 Employers in industry, commerce, etc. (small establishments)
3.   Professional workers – self-employed
4.   Professional workers – employees
5.1 Intermediate non-manual workers – ancillary workers and artists
5.2 Intermediate non-manual workers – foremen and supervisors non-manual
6.   Junior non-manual workers
7.   Personal service workers
8.   Foremen and supervisors – manual
9.   Skilled manual workers
10. Semi-skilled manual workers
11. Unskilled manual workers
12. Own-account workers (other than professional)
13. Farmers – employers and managers
14. Farmers – own account
15. Agricultural workers
16. Members of armed forces
17. Inadequately described and not stated occupations

(Adapted from Rose and Pevalin, 2005, p7)

However, this has been subject to criticism as being inadequately sensitive for contemporary statistical analysis and for capturing the inadequacies of the state in providing equal access to health, education, housing and employment, so a further classification model has been developed.

Operational categories of the National Statistics: Socio-economic Classification (NS-SEC)

L1 Employers in large establishments
L2 Higher managerial occupations
L3 Higher professional occupations
    L3.1 'Traditional' employees
    L3.2 'New' employees
    L3.3 'Traditional' self-employed
    L3.4 'New' self-employed

L4   Lower professional and higher technical occupations
    L4.1   'Traditional' employees
    L4.2   'New' employees
    L4.3   'Traditional' self-employed
    L4.4   'New' self-employed
L5   Lower managerial occupations
L6   Higher supervisory occupations
L7   Intermediate occupations
    L7.1   Intermediate clerical and administrative occupations
    L7.2   Intermediate service occupations
    L7.3   Intermediate technical and auxiliary occupations
    L7.4   Intermediate engineering occupations
L8   Employers in small organisations
    L8.1   Employers in small organisations in industry, commerce, services, etc.
    L8.2   Employers in small organisations in agriculture
L9   Own-account workers
    L9.1   Own-account workers (non-professional)
    L9.2   Own-account workers in agriculture
L10 Lower supervisory occupations
L11 Lower technical occupations
    L11.1   Lower technical craft occupations
    L11.2   Lower technical process operative occupations
L12 Semi-routine occupations
    L12.1   Semi-routine sales occupations
    L12.2   Semi-routine service occupations
    L12.3   Semi-routine technical occupations
    L12.4   Semi-routine operative occupations
    L12.5   Semi-routine agricultural occupations
    L12.6   Semi-routine clerical occupations
    L12.7   Semi-routine childcare occupations
L13 Routine occupations
    L13.1   Routine sales and service occupations
    L13.2   Routine production occupations
    L13.3   Routine technical occupations
    L13.4   Routine operative occupations
    L13.5   Routine agricultural occupations
L14 Never worked and long-term unemployed
    L14.2   Long-term unemployed
L15 Full-time students
L16 Occupations not stated or inadequately described
L17 Not classifiable for other reasons

(Adapted from Rose and Pevalin, 2005, p17)

The historical development of these classification systems indicates the increasing complexity of the structure of our society. For a full discussion and report on the current classification system used by the ONS, see Rose and Pevalin (2005).

Politically and sociologically, class differentials have been the subject of much debate and continue to be used to delineate social divisions in society and the distribution of wealth. The impact of social origins on life chances continues to be researched (Platt, 2005). The gap in the share of income between the richest and the poorest has increased, and also employment and educational achievements continue to be determined by social background (Devine et al., 2004). Added to this are economic changes that are affecting society, such as the decrease in traditional working-class employment in the manufacturing industry and the increase in the service industry. The development of the welfare state in the twentieth century is held to be responsible for a broader middle-class grouping and the emergence of other categories, such as gender and ethnicity, which are competing with class distinctions as having an effect on life's chances.

The implication for nursing is that we are expected to work with persons from all aspects of life and, when communicating with persons from different socio-economic backgrounds, it is important not to make assumptions based upon class stereotypes. People move from one group to another and can be affected by a variety of circumstances. There is a danger that collusion can occur between similar groups and issues can be overlooked, for example, middle-class health visitors overlooking child abuse in middle-class families. The use of restricted language should not be confused with levels of comprehension. All patients are entitled to full explanations of their treatments and interventions in a manner that is helpful and neutral from assumptions, for example that the most educated do not need explanations and those with less education need more, or that people with mental health problems do not need to be routinely informed about the short- and long-term side-effects of their prescribed medications. It is the clarity and quality of the explanation that is relevant and everyone needs reassurance, regardless of their socio-economic position (see Chapter 5).

Race and culture

The UK has a population that is composed of a wide variety of cultures, religions and languages. There are over 100 different languages spoken in London schools. While there are differing concentrations of multiculturalism throughout the four countries, the UK is no longer a white homogeneous nation. To think so is to devalue the minority cultures within our society and disregard aspects of people's lives. This denial can lead to racist attitudes and can act as a barrier to good practice in healthcare. Communication and interpersonal interactions need to be ethnically sensitive and anti-racist. Assumptions, for example on skin colour determining biological differences, have the potential to be used as arguments for the destructive mythology of racial inferiority. Taking the time to understand cultural and ethnic beliefs and practices is needed, as well as listening to the stories of friends and colleagues who have been harassed or abused through racism – if they trust you enough to share their experiences.

Gender

From a normative perspective (Zeeman et al., 2014b), there is an acknowledgement of recognisable differences between men and women in most societies, and a corresponding male/female divide that has various codes and expectations of behaviour and responses in social interaction. From this perspective, by the age of two, infants can recognise the differences through hair and clothes, aided by significant gender stereotyping that is prevalent in most societies. The extent to which gender differences are innate or learned is, though, the subject of debate. To complicate matters further, the apparently straightforward binary divide between 'male' and 'female' has been challenged by contemporary theoretical and empirical work on health and healthcare (Zeeman et al., 2014b). Social constructionists, such as Burr (2003), claim that gender is constructed through everyday discourse and reinforced through communication patterns, whereas evolutionary theorists argue that gender variations in behaviour arise only from biological differences. The jury is still out, but there seems a strong case for both nature and nurture to play a role in varying degrees.

Studies of gender-related communication behaviours suggest that women prefer less interpersonal space, that they touch and are touched more, gesture less, look and are looked at more and smile more frequently. Social skills inventories have revealed consistent gender differences on various dimensions, females scoring higher on measures of emotional expressivity and sensitivity (Hargie, 2006). Males prefer to be more directive, self-opinionated and explicit, whereas females tend to be more indirect, use a greater number of uncertainties ('it could be'; 'might be'), that is, passive speech styles, speak for longer periods and refer more to emotions.

There are inconsistencies in the studies reporting these behaviours and the general view is that gender is something we 'do' rather than something we 'are'.

The development of feminism and the critical feminist movement has helped to widen our understanding of women's place in society and the contribution they make. There remain concerns over the unequal distribution of power and life chances between men and women. To overcome these concerns there continues to be a need to retain a critical view of how women are treated in healthcare settings to ensure that their needs are not overlooked and that male dominance is not reinforced or legitimised. It is important to ensure that women's problems are constructed in women's terms and not men's, and that stereotypical gender expectations are challenged if they are without evidence or foundation. There are specific examples of female-related health problems (for example, sexual abuse and depression) that may pass unnoticed unless highlighted.

Men can also experience problems associated with sexism when rigid stereotyping expects certain responses from them around how they are expected to think, feel and act. This is particularly evident at times of bereavement.

When men and women interact within a context of gender inequality, barriers to communication and interpersonal relationships can inhibit effective assessment and health interventions. The danger is that gender inequality can exacerbate or reinforce existing problems (for example, low self-esteem) and lack of opportunity to speak, describe or express ideas on problems that are being presented. The prevailing advice is to assume a neutral communication style and be aware of using your own gender stereotypical behaviour in interactions.

Sexual orientation

Taking the biological view that sexuality is purely, or primarily, a biological phenomenon, and heterosexuality deemed to be natural and normal, inevitably defines homosexuality as unnatural and abnormal. This view, however, rules out those in society who have an alternative sexual orientation. The social and psychological dimensions of sexuality are relevant in this discussion as they provide explanations for an alternative view of sexuality that cannot be ignored or marginalised. If not considered, the only concept of sexuality is based on heteronormative assumptions, and is limited to the biological argument, reinforcing the potential to lead to misunderstandings, prejudice and discrimination (Zeeman et al., 2014b).

It has to be acknowledged that gay and lesbian relationships, which are accepted in some cultures, are not in others. In many countries, same-sex couples could face severe punishment or death, whereas in other countries they can be recognised legally. This creates an additional dilemma for health professionals who, on the one hand, are prepared to help persons regardless of their sexual orientation, but who, on the other hand, will also take into account the beliefs of persons in their care that may not, through reasons of faith or culture, accept homosexuality. Nurses may also have their own cultural beliefs, which could be challenged by this situation. As with other diverse groups under discussion, respect, fairness and dignity are important features of working in a professional and non-judgemental manner, and are the precepts to be guided by in these encounters in the healthcare context.

Communication with members of the trans communities

It is important to be aware that 'gender identity' is separate from sexual orientation. Sexual orientation refers to the gender or genders that someone is sexually attracted to, whereas gender identity refers to the ways in which a person describes how they experience themselves with regard to the gender they embody. The word 'trans' is an umbrella term. It is used to describe people whose sex/gender diverges in some ways from the sex/gender assigned to them at birth, and to transgendered men and women who seek treatment and surgical interventions to modify their bodies. However it is also used to refer to people who live outside of dominant gender norms without seeking surgical interventions. Some trans people identify as heterosexual, some as LGBQUI (lesbian, gay, bisexual, queer, undecided or intersex), whereas others may refuse sexual and/or gender categorization or language which attempts to describe or define this. The trans communities therefore include the following groups of people (note that this is not an exhaustive or definitive list):

Transgender, transsexual, genderqueer, intersex, non-binary, bi-gender, genderfluid, cross-dresser, trans man, trans women, and agender.

Activity 7.4   *Critical thinking*

Individually, explore the meanings of all of the above terms, in relation to 'cisgender', 'heteronormativity' and 'homonormativity'.

Then in groups, discuss the implications emerging for the professional relationships between nurses and those who would regard themselves as members of the trans communities, which will include clients, patients, users, survivors, relatives and other nurses and healthcare staff, around:

- The choice of personal pronouns that trans individuals might want to be represented by, verbally and in writing (eg 'he', 'she', 'they').
- The tensions that a nurse might find themselves in with regard to the above, between medico-legal practices and constraints and the freedom of representational self-representation at an individual level.

Now read Aramburu Alegria C (2011) Transgender identity and health care: Implications for psychosocial and physical evaluation. *Journal of the American Academy of Nurse Practitioners*, 23: 175–182. Discuss this paper in groups.

Hint: Engaging in all of these activities will better sensitise you to the need to exercise sensitivity in interpersonal relationships with these groups of people.

We live in times where sexuality does not coincide with gender, where neither sexuality nor gender are always clear categories for capturing people's experiences and behaviour, and thus where traditional binaries for describing people – 'man', 'woman', heterosexual', 'homosexual' – are often and arguably increasingly regarded as inadequate and sometimes inappropriate. Prosser (2013, p34), for example, recently described 'trans' as an 'incessant destablizing movement between sexual and gender identities', signalling one of the overall aims and functions of Queer scholarship in disrupting and troubling binaried identities (Zeeman et al., 2014a, b).

In her generally important resource for practice, Arambura Alegria (2011, p179) argued that it is important to address 'transgender persons in a gender-appropriate manner'. She went on to argue on the basis of this assertion that persons who have transitioned from male to female should be addressed as women and, conversely, persons who have transitioned from female to male should be addressed as men. This may indeed seem, and often be, an appropriate courtesy strategy for nurses to adopt. However, Arambura Alegria's advice here may yet be regarded as presumptious and inappropriate by some transgendered patients, clients, service users or mental health survivors. This is because of the fluidity of identity and related self-referential terms highlighted in both the list of possible categories and the Queer scholarship described above. Thus, tact, sensitivity and checking out with people on the use of personal pronouns and gender-related descriptive language are crucial first steps in establishing good interpersonal relationships in these cultural contexts.

Age

Ageism is a term generally applied to discrimination against older persons, although it can be applied to children. When applied to older persons it can be characterised by a number of factors.

- *Marginalisation* – older people and their needs are rarely seen as a priority or a central concern.
- *Dehumanisation* – older people are represented as 'over the hill' and of little use to society.
- *Infantalisation* – older people tend to be treated like children, for example by using first names, or nicknames, without asking the person if this is acceptable.

The phenomenon of social ageing, or how we behave in social encounters towards each other, and our understanding of the differences between ourselves and others as we age or change are thought to be achieved through communication. Our own age, and the ages of those with whom we interact, shape our responses, behaviours and expectations. Therefore, we take the target of our responses into consideration and frame them accordingly. So, for example, a reward for a child would be 'You're a clever little person', for an adolescent 'You have really grown up' and for an older person it could be 'I find your ideas very interesting'. Adapting to make the apposite response is how we reduce ageism and at the same time guard against being patronising.

Reaction times, speech recognition and the capacity for information processing slow down with ageing; however, this happens at a different rate for different individuals. Older people have often had years of experience in dealing with people from different backgrounds and in different situations, and have gained a wealth of language to use in these contexts. Regrettably, there is negative stereotyping for the older person that is transformed into the use of secondary baby talk, elderspeak and patronising talk. This is often the result of intentions to be helpful, such as slowing down or simplification of messages and clarification exercises, for example raising the volume of the voice, deliberate articulation and diminutives such as 'dear' or 'love'. These patterns, as well as being demeaning, have a negative effect on the self-identity of elderly persons and reinforce their sense of loss of control and dependency.

The implications for the nurse are to consider pitching responses at the apposite level, having first assessed the ability (rather than chronological age) of the other person. There is also a danger of concentrating on the physical needs of older people and not considering their rights or choices.

Disability

Disability is often viewed as a physical problem that stands in the way of normal social functioning. An alternative view is that social attitudes to disability are the disabling function rather than the impairment itself. An example of this is that it is not the use of a wheelchair that bars access to buildings; it is the lack of disabled access and a ramp that causes the disability. The social model of disability draws attention to the tendency of disabled people to be marginalised, dehumanised and patronised (there are similarities here to ageism). There is a focus on limitations rather than potential and capability. There is also a lack of awareness of the barriers, both physical and attitudinal, that prevent disabled persons from becoming integrated into society. Finally, there is a tendency to focus on dependency rather than empowerment (Oliver, 1990).

Here are some suggestions for interpersonal communication concerning disabilities (adapted from DeVito, 2007).

- Avoid negative terms and terms that define the person as disabled, such as 'the disabled man' or 'the handicapped child'.

- Instead, say 'person with a disability', always emphasising the person rather than the disability. Avoid describing the person with a disability as 'abnormal'; when you define people without disabilities as 'normal', you say, in effect, that the person with the disability isn't normal.

- Treat assistive devices such as wheelchairs, canes, walkers or crutches as the personal property of the user. Don't move these out of your way; they're for the convenience of the person with the disability. Avoid leaning on a person's wheelchair – it is similar to leaning on the person.

- Shake hands with the person with the disability if you shake hands with others in the group. Don't avoid shaking hands because the individual's hand is disfigured or misshapen, for example.

- Avoid talking about the person with a disability in the third person. For example, avoid saying 'Doesn't he get around beautifully with the new crutches?' Direct your comments to the individual.

- Don't assume that people who have a disability are intellectually impaired. Slurred speech, such as may occur with cerebral palsy or cleft palate, should never be taken as indicating a low-level intellect. So be especially careful not to talk down to people, as many do.

- When you're not sure of how to act, ask. For example, if you're not sure if you should offer walking assistance, say 'Would you like me to help you into the dining room?' And, more importantly, accept the person's response. If he or she says no, then that means no! So don't insist.

- Maintain similar eye level. If the person is in a wheelchair, for example, it might be helpful for you to sit down or kneel down to maintain the same eye level.

Ethical and moral dimensions

Because there are consequences of communication and personal interactions, whether deliberate or unintentional, there are also ethical considerations to take into account. Each communication situation has a moral dimension of rightness and wrongness, where the expectation is that communication will be honest, decent, just and appropriate. These moral principles are often expected and implicit in interactions. There is an expectation that nurses will respect individuals and act within the NMC *Code of Professional Conduct* (2004b), which embodies these principles. Within a cultural context, these have to be considered and interpreted according to the respective value systems of each culture. An example is the close physical proximity in which much nursing takes place, which creates an additional layer of ethical complexity, related to intimacy, as discussed previously in Chapter 2. There are many occasions when decisions and choices about healthcare treatments and therapies have to be guided by ethical considerations, as well as concerns about the effectiveness of a chosen path and the satisfaction this will give to the patients and carers.

A first step towards making decisions that take account of cultural variability is to understand the way in which culture influences how health and illness are understood by the members of a cultural group or community sharing the same values. The cultural interpretation of health and illness is based upon values and perceptions that are the product of the combination of traditions, lived experiences and the knowledge sanctioned by a particular culture. The values are often derived from the notion of health as a resource – how this features in daily lives and how this affects the productivity, effectiveness, significance and status of people in their community.

The dominant framework for understanding the cause and treatment of ill health in the western world is the **biomedical model**. The conceptual framework for the biomedical model is that illness is caused by the malfunctioning of a specific bodily part and the part in question needs to be treated so that the illness may be removed. The emphasis is on cure, often technical and/or pharmacological, which is based upon the broader scientific notions of control through empirical observation and driven by evidence from controlled experiments or studies. The assumption is that the model provides a truthful account of reality when compared to more primitive forms of healing and curing practices, which are not empirically based and hence irrational. The model has relevance in delivering effective solutions in certain instances; however, it is not culturally sensitive.

Case study: A complex interaction of responses

Alisha is 42 years old and works as a cleaner in an office building in a large UK city. She came to the UK from West Bengal, India, 22 years ago as a young bride. She barely makes a living and depends upon her work to supplement her husband's wages and support her family of five children, two of whom are adults but unemployed and living at home. In discussing her health, Alisha reveals a complex interaction of responses. If she considers the illness to be very serious she will go to the local hospital, even though she knows she will have to wait a long time to be seen and it will be difficult to explain to the nurses and doctors why she is there, because her English is limited. This is the last resort. For persistent fevers in her children she will go to the local allopathic doctor (using remedies whose effects differ from those produced by the disease), even though there will be high fees to pay, because she will not have to wait. In other instances, she may visit the homeopathic doctor, who is more affordable. She will also visit the kobiraj (the Ayurvedic practitioner). Finally, while Alisha knows that allopathic medicine will offer relief, she knows it will not cure. For this to happen, Alisha believes the underlying causes have to be dealt with and these are connected to divine forces. To solve this problem, Alisha makes offerings at the temple of the goddess Kali so that she will be appeased.

This case study gives an example of the centrality of culture in the perception of health and illness. It also illuminates the different resources and organisational structures that individuals may resort to for solutions to health problems. The notion of a divine origin of health, and models other than the biomedical utilised by Alisha to understand the cause and cure of illness, indicate a complex terrain of a cultural space where health and illness are negotiated.

Case study: Exploring alternatives

Jane, a single woman, was diagnosed with breast cancer at the age of 43. Even though Jane, who works as a hospital secretary, had good relationships with medical and nursing staff and had faith in their abilities, she decided to explore other treatment options. She surfed the internet for articles and gathered feedback from her friends and family. The most common response she found was, 'have it removed'. She thought this was good advice and made an appointment for surgery. As the date approached, she became more and more unsure. She read more articles that questioned the efficacy of surgery and she found alternative suggestions. These ranged from yoga to meditation and guided imagery. She was thinking of delaying the surgery and her friends advised her that she was losing precious time, yet she felt that the alternative approaches had more meaning for her.

Activity 7.5   *Decision making*

List the differences and similarities between the two cases above.

• What is the prevailing similarity and the most significant difference and can these be reconciled in the healthcare system we have in the UK? Can you describe the cultural origins of these two cases without stereotyping?
• What can be learned from the second case, and the health decisions and choices Jane has to make when she navigates the healthcare system? If you were Jane's friend, how would you advise her? Would this be different from the advice you would give as a professional? What are the moral obligations you have as a professional?

Hint: Think of evidence-based practice, and your role as an advocate. This activity is aimed to help you develop your critical abilities around culturally sensitive, ethical decision making. In order to minimise stereotyping, use only the facts before you.

Alisha's story involves shifting from one form of treatment to another depending on the nature of the illness, the location of the person in the family structure, the price and the time it takes to receive treatment and transport. These options are interwoven into a complex web of meaning involving hierarchies and resources. The treatments lie outside the biomedical model as well as engage with it, indicating a crossroads between a culture-centred approach and a biomedical approach. Here is a nexus for ethical decision making using communication skills that enable a deeper understanding of cultural values and issues.

Chapter summary

In this chapter we have considered the extent to which our population is changing and the need for increased understanding and awareness of multicultural needs in health-care. We have also explored the definitions of culture and have discussed the socio-economic factors impacting upon today's healthcare recipients. As well as considering the diverse population needs of groups in society in relation to socio-economic position, race and culture, gender, sexual orientation, age and disability, we have examined the ethical and moral dimensions of communication and interpersonal relationships in a culturally diverse world.

Further reading

Clarke, V, Ellis, SJ, Peel, E and Riggs, DW (2010) *Lesbian, Gay, Bisexual, Trans and Queer Psychology: An introduction.* Cambridge: Cambridge University Press.

Dutte, MJ (2008) *Communicating Health: A culture-centred approach.* Cambridge: Polity Press.
This book explores health communication from the perspective of culture.

Prosser, J (2013) Judith Butler: queer feminism, transgender, and the transubstantiation of sex. In: Hall, DE, Jagose, A, with Bebell, A and Potter, S (eds) *The Routledge Queer Studies Reader.* London and New York: Routledge.

Zeeman, L, Aranda, K and Grant, A (2014) *Queering Health: Critical challenges to normative health and Healthcare.* Ross-on-Wye: PCCS Books.
The above books will help you explore in greater depth the interpersonal and communication implications related to working with trans populations.

Useful websites

http://www.ons.gov.uk/ons/guide-method/census/2011/index.html
This website contains information on the National Census.

http://www.ons.gov.uk/ons/guide-method/classifications/current-standard-classifications/soc2010/soc2010-volume-3-ns-sec–rebased-on-soc2010–user-manual/index.html
Here you will find details of the National Statistics Socio-economic Classification.

http://www.ons.gov.uk/ons/taxonomy/index.html?nscl=International+Migration
This website gives information on immigration and migration.

http://www.womenshealthresearch.org
This is the website for the Society for Women's Health Research.

www.lgbtnetwork.eu
The website of the LGBT network.

www.clareproject.org.uk/home/support/support-resources
The Clare Project booklet *So, Someone You Know is Transgender, Questions and Answers for Family, Friends and Colleagues* is available on this website.

Chapter 8
Beyond technique

Chapter aims

By the end of this chapter, in relation to the increasingly skilled practice of CIPS, you should be able to:

- understand the differences between **professional artistry** and **technical rationality** at theoretical and applied levels;
- describe what is meant by **critical reflexivity**;
- outline the place of critical reflexivity in the tensions between professional artistry and technical rationality in nursing;
- understand the significance of these tensions in the development of compassion in organisations;
- describe the place and significance of critical reflexivity in healthcare organisational development.

Introduction

Having got this far in your reading of the book, we now want to take you in this concluding chapter to a place 'beyond technique'. This place is not explicitly linked to NMC competencies or Essential Skills Clusters because it speaks to issues that are broader, deeper and arguably more profound than can be adequately captured in contemporary nursing policy. Our purpose in doing this is to help you think more critically about your future in terms of the developing and unending practice of, and engagement with, the complexities of skilled interpersonal practice.

Your initial thought might be that the title of this chapter is a little strange; that 'CIPS in nursing' is surely all about technique! In some respects, this is of course true. However, the conscientious practice of CIPS in nursing which begins for you as a self-conscious endeavour should, over time, move you to a point where such practice becomes internalised as an increasingly refined automatic skills set. Equipped with this, you will hopefully and ideally do the right interpersonal thing at the appropriate time, without thinking too much about it. Moreover, as you know by now, the skilled practice of CIPS does not take place in a contextual vacuum, so it is important to understand that this skills set will link to, and be informed by, multiple knowledge sources.

This chapter will help you, therefore, to move forward in this journey in relation to a number of interlinked contexts, within which you will be able to situate CIPS in nursing within professional developmental, cultural, social-organisational, political and moral concerns. Specifically, you will be invited to consider:

165

- the context of CIPS in professional development at the level of *professional artistry* (Polanyi, 1967; Schön, 1987);

- how such professional artistry can be further understood at *critically reflexive* levels of increased organisational and political awareness (Freshwater and Rolfe, 2001);

- how all of this links to the culture of contemporary nursing practice in terms of how the professional artistry paradigm (world-view) is in tension with the paradigm of *technical rationality* (Schön, 1987), and the political implications for nursing practice that emerge from this tension;

- how this developing complexity of CIPS in nursing practice has further implications for the social organisation of healthcare practice, with regard to how nurses relate to each other, to other healthcare staff, and to patients, clients, service users and carers, within their practice organisations;

- how exclusively technical rational approaches to CIPS in nursing practice may arguably undermine, trivialise and debase their worth;

- finally, how many healthcare organisational members may be blind to this, underscoring the importance of critical reflexivity (Morgan, 2006; Alvesson and Spicer, 2012).

Towards professional artistry in CIPS

The shift from self-conscious practice to skilled reflexive practice is an important transition journey for nurses, who, as has been vigorously argued throughout this book, all need to demonstrate increasing finesse in the area of interpersonal communication and relationships. In terms of professional development, this shift represents the move from what Schön (1987) described as the practice of technical rationality to the artistry of the professional practice of CIPS. All practising nurses who persevere in the lifelong endeavour to improve on their understanding and practice of CIPS will draw professional artistry from the embodied reservoir of what Polanyi (1967) called *tacit knowledge*. This term refers to knowledge resources held by skilled nurses that are not easily made explicit or codified in language. Nurses draw on these resources flexibly in myriad different contexts, and act on them in automatic rather than deliberate and thought-through ways.

Theory summary: Professional artistry

Schön (1987) argued that those who practise, or advocate practice, at the level of technical rationality see the world in terms of *well-formed instrumental problems* (pp3–4) which require *specific technique* solutions. However, as most seasoned nursing professionals know, this model of the world of practice can be criticised for beeing simplistic and one-dimensional. Most nursing clinical scenarios requiring skilled CIPS practice are messy and complex. So, attempts to reduce them to the level of straightforward 'one problem, one right solution' are doomed to fail.

Polanyi (1967) described the remarkable, embodied virtuosity with which we recognise and do the right thing in an immediate way, without being too aware of our reasoning processes that lead up to this, or engaging in a laboured comparison of the action we choose to take with alternatives. So, one consequence of becoming skilful in the area of CIPS in nursing is to learn to exercise appropriate action directly, in the absence of intermediate reasoning.

As an aspirational goal, professional artistry has long been recognised as crucial in advancing interpersonal work in the helping professions, through helping practitioners develop along a continuum from novice to expert practice. For example, this is promoted in all nursing by Benner (1982, 2000) and specifically in specialist mental health and mental health nurse psychotherapeutic practice by Grant (2010a).

Professional artistry and critical reflexivity

By this stage in the book, you should be familiar with the argument for the importance of reflective practice in professional nursing. Freshwater and Rolfe (2001) argued that professional artistry, which in Schön's (1987) terms is developed through the process of *reflection-in-action* (or how our thinking helps us reshape what we are doing *while we are doing it*) should also involve the exercise of critical reflexivity. The practice of critical reflexivity takes us beyond personal introspection to demand that we are forever mindful of the social and political contexts in which our CIPS practice takes place.

Activity 8.1	*Research and reflection*

Read Freshwater, D and Rolfe, G (2001) Critical reflexivity: a politically and ethically engaged research method for nursing. *NT Research*, 6(1): 526–537.

Available online at:

http://garyrolfe.net/documents/criticalreflexivity.pdf

In a small group, discuss the implications emerging from this article for CIPS nursing practice.

Clearly, relationships – whether between nurses and other healthcare professionals, or between nurses and clients, patients, service users, survivors or carers – do not take place in an organisational vacuum. We have already learned from earlier chapters that environmental and other structural forces shape the nature of relationships in many ways.

This is an important issue, and gives the lie to the kinds of 'quick-fix' interpersonal solutions that belong to a decontextualised, technical-rational view of nursing. At all levels, nursing is political (taking place within power relationships), historically contingent (taking place at particular points in time, with associated policy and public perception demands on how nursing is perceived and practised) and socially and environmentally contextual (taking place within specific configurations of relationships, events and work settings). This overall state of affairs will inevitably place demands on you to embrace critical reflexivity, in order to develop your professional artistry of CIPS within the messiness of the contradictions that constitute real-life nursing practice and contemporary healthcare cultures. In this regard, it is important to be mindful of the fact that fundamental to the moral and ethical dimensions of professional artistry is the need to be human rather than mechanical.

Activity 8.2	*Critical thinking*

Some contradictions within competing narratives of the meaning and function of compassionate nursing

With fellow students, discuss the following argument, presented from different perspectives. One perspective is that CIPS skills can be taught on the basis of a simple rote learning, or algorithmic, model to combat compassion deficits in healthcare. This is challenged by critical social science perspectives. The argument focuses on the question: is the technical-rational assumption of CIPS as a set of skills that can be taught in a context-neutral way sufficient to remedy major interpersonal problems between nurses and the people in their care?

In response to the mid-Staffordshire and other scandals, some NHS Trusts are currently and understandably commissioning 'compassion teaching'. The assumption is that such teaching will play a significant part in reducing the likelihood of future large-scale interpersonal assaults by nurses and other healthcare workers on the people they are supposed to be caring for. How realistic is it, however, to expect that compassion skills teaching will make a major contribution to sustained, large-scale and meaningful improvements to nursing practice while the politico-economic structures that arguably gave rise to them in the first place remain relatively unchanged?

From a critical, Marxist perspective (Newton et al., 1995), an over-emphasis on nurses taking individual responsibility to develop compassion skills arguably does little to address the economic, structural and cultural problems that contribute significantly to the emergence of patterns of wide-scale abuse. In this regard, individualising interpersonal and other abuses at the levels of problem (abusive nurses constitute 'a few bad apples') and solution (if nurses are taught correctly, they are more likely to choose to practise correctly) seems simplistic and flawed.

In complementary terms, from a social psychological perspective, Zimbardo (2009) argues that relatively unchanging politico-economic structures are likely ultimately to militate against individualised good intentions. This is because the contemporary culture of organisational performance- and target-driven public services (Seddon, 2008), which contributed greatly to the emergence of the Mid-Staffordshire and other abuses, still hold sway and thus function as powerful shapers of the behaviour of health workers.

The proposition is that cultures that shape nursing professional identity at levels of healthcare custom, practice and assumptions are forever likely to undermine the best efforts and intentions of human agency to produce large-scale and lasting change for the better in healthcare organisational practice. In politico-economic conditions that privilege organisational efficiency around systems, targets, control and compliance, empathic human relating will be accorded relatively less respect, despite policy and educational rhetoric.

Building on the argument of Chapter 1 of the power of environments to shape experiences and behaviour, different healthcare work settings will clearly have varying impact on the type, extent and level of empathic human relating that is possible in each. However, if the argument developing in this chapter is accepted, technical-rational principles cannot be intelligently regarded as sufficient in providing a blanket solution to CIPS problems in environments that are culturally and structurally antagonistic to such practice. Consider to what extent the following case study illustrates one such example of this from the private healthcare sector.

Case study

In September 2014, the magazine Private Eye *(no. 1374, p32) reported that a care worker in a private nursing home had been ostracised at work for several weeks, after complaining to her managers about residents suffering because there were too few staff to care for them properly. She described how she had been taunted by chants of 'loose lips sink ships' and expressed that she felt she was being driven out of her job. However she was positive about her intention to turn out for a demonstration to be held outside parliament in late September 2014 of carers, health workers and relatives of those who have suffered neglect and poor care, who are lobbying for urgent reform of the law to protect whistleblowers (see Compassion in Care website at the bottom of this chapter).*

Being skilled is not the same as being kind

Technical-rational competence in CIPS does not necessarily and simply equate to being compassionate on the basis of universal understandings of kindness (Phillips and Taylor, 2009). It may be instructive to consider this assertion in relation to what some nurse scholars describe as an international picture of nursing higher education curricula biased strongly in favour of competency development (Shields et al., 2012). If this picture is accepted then, ironically, it may follow that CIPS competencies serve to conceal the absence of kindness in many practice areas, whereas critically reflexive learning might result in exposing this.

Clearly healthcare environments need to support such learning if it is to result in a better standard of CIPS practice. In this regard, it has been argued that critically reflexive professionals may often be perceived as a threat to the smooth running of such organisations, given their tendency to challenge fundamental organisational procedural assumptions (Grant, 2014b). However, if the status quo of healthcare practice around CIPS is to be engaged with, scrutinised and improved, so that the people in our care and the colleagues we work with are treated more compassionately and kindly, it seems axiomatic that we need the presence of outspoken, critically reflexive practitioners in our healthcare and related services.

This message is strongly endorsed by Crawford (2014, p1), who makes the incisive point that the advances in technology informing contemporary nursing work, which relate to the need for competency-driven educational practices:

serve principally as a means of treating more patients, and are mainly used to get the conveyor belt they travel on to go faster [with the] . . . metrics, targets and production-line methologies that have come to dominate our way of thinking.

In this context, international higher education practices understandably and necessarily follow such advances in the aim of producing nursing practitioners who are both competency-savvy and competency-skilled (Shields et al., 2012). However, enabling nursing to practise in such ways, although valued by healthcare organisations, may also contribute to undermining the development of professional artistry in nursing CIPS. This is because 'blip culture' encounters (Toffler, 1980; Brown et al., 2006), limited to a few minutes or less, may be all that is possible or, indeed, regarded as important in many contemporary, competency-focused practice environments which operate according to technical-rational principles.

Activity 8.3   *Team working*

Discuss the following proposition with your peers:

Frequently, nurses may 'say the right things' to patients/clients/service users, their relatives and carers, or colleagues, only for their facial expressions to give the lie to, and contradict, their words. The net result of this is that such nurses may at best appear shallow, patronising and/or insensitive, and at worst downright disingenuous. This phenomenon does not just apply to a small minority of nurses, since the need for human beings generally to engage in *impression management* (Goffman, 1959) is likely to mean that in pressurised, competency- rather than relationally-led, work situations the motivation to be convincingly seen to 'perform' compassion may simultaneously undermine such performance. Thus, attempts to disseminate CIPS knowledge and practice, solely based on a focus on events such as 'compassionate awareness' sessions, and humanising nursing, may amount to two different and contradictory projects that relate to each other in antagonistic ways. From a skills training perspective, 'compassionate' nursing behaviour may remain brittle and palpably false, hidden behind a veneer of professionalism, CIPS models and algorithms, which are more coldly efficient rather than, in terms of kindness, compassionate in humane and heartfelt ways (Baker, 2013).

Hint: There is no one right way to approach the above discussion exercise. It is simply intended to help you work through and consider some of its points in dialogue with others.

Critical theory: The practice of CIPS in nursing

The mechanical practice of CIPS in nursing links to technical-rational assumptions about its need to be taught in relation to the perceived potential or actual insufficiency of compassion in healthcare organisations. This links in turn to a response to the emergence in the 1970s and 1980s of a lack of trust in public services discourse. According to the moral philosopher Onora O'Neill (2002), this lack of trust resulted in healthcare and other public service organisations aiming for public 'transparency' through micro-management while actually creating cultures of deception. In this regard, Seddon (2008) argues that contemporary target-driven public service work cultures are frequently focused more on the need for public impression management and risk avoidance than fulfilling their care and treatment functions in morally coherent ways. In other words, many public-sector organisational cultures may be more concerned about how their services, and the people within them, look than about what they do or how well they do it.

The critically reflexive nurse as organisational role model

The argument in this chapter so far places a demand on contemporary nurses to strive towards functioning as critically reflexive CIPS role models, to challenge technologically and competency-sanctioned bad practice, and related, organisational norms around unsatisfactory interpersonal relationships. In short, nurses should role-model humanness; we need to practise what we preach.

However, there are many ways in which CIPS-challenged organisations will mirror the poor and unsatisfactory relationships between staff members that, when experienced by patients and their relatives, result in complaints and the exposure of abusive practices. Ironically and tragically underscoring the need for nurses to strive towards ever greater levels of critically reflexive sophistication, CIPS-challenged organisations will often not be recognised as such by many of their members, who will employ the kinds of organisational defence mechanisms described earlier in this book to protect themselves from such awareness (Morgan, 2006).

In this regard, Alvesson and Spicer (2012) argue that a feature of the kinds of bureaucratic organisations we work in is *functional stupidity*. This term refers to a cognitively and emotionally informed unwillingness or inability to employ reflexivity or frank discussion about assumptions and related practice embedded in organisations. Thus many nurses and their managers are likely instead to regard the behaviours and experiences listed below as 'perfectly reasonable business as usual'.

Characteristics of the CIPS-challenged organisation

CIPS-challenged organisations are characterised by some or all of the following (and this list is by no means comprehensive: try adding to it):

- staff not really involved in decision making, despite organisational rhetoric suggesting the opposite;
- managers expecting healthcare staff to attend CIPS-related and other seminars and training, but viewing their own attendance as irrelevant or unnecessary;
- staff finding themselves in 'I–it' rather than 'I–thou' relationships (Buber, 1958) (see Chapter 1), by, for example, being told how they are feeling or what they should be doing rather than being invited into dialogue about this;
- colleagues and managers violating the principle of turn taking in conversations at meetings, through constant interruptions, with multiple people talking at once, while demonstrating a failure to listen to the person who has the floor at any particular point in the meeting;

- staff receiving blip culture e-mails that are both confusing through an over-use of unexplained acronyms and lacking in necessary context, which thus do not contain (and indeed may obscure) the necessary vital information for them to reply appropriately and in an informed way;

- staff feeling compromised as a result of vital information not being passed on (to the ultimate disadvantage of patients);

- senior staff and colleagues not responding to e-mails, or responding long after the need for a response has passed, thus trivialising the concerns of the sender of the original e-mail;

- senior staff being perpetually unavailable for contact with junior staff, by maintaining a 'closed-door' style, or restricting contact through managing interpersonal contact solely by time slot appointment or bureaucratic diktat;

- senior staff constantly trivialising the concerns of more junior staff verbally, or even ignoring their physical presence;

- staff being expected to account for themselves in a hurried way, in blip culture encounters, within which considered and patient discussion of context is sacrificed to 'bullet point' dialogues and exchanges;

- colleagues failing to display normal civil courtesies, for example in exchanging smiles or verbal acknowledgements when they pass each other in corridors, or doing so in curt, dismissive or cold ways.

Activity 8.4 *Team working*

Informally survey your peers and practice colleagues, to gauge the extent to which they identify or disagree with any of the bullet points listed immediately above. If they connect with any, ask them how this leaves them feeling. Conversely, if they disagree with any, ask them how they experience their organisation as different. In both cases, reflect upon the ways in which their responses might relate to how patients, clients or service users are regarded and treated in the healthcare organisations they work in.

Chapter summary

This chapter began by contextualising CIPS for each nurse in a developing professional artistry underpinned by organisationally and politically aware critical reflexivity. The discussion moved on to how professional artistry may be threatened by technical rationality in contemporary nursing practice. This was shown to have implications for the relationships between and among nurses and other healthcare staff and between nurses and the people in their care. It was argued that exclusively technical-rational approaches to CIPS in nursing practice may undermine, trivialise and debase its worth. Finally, the importance of critical reflexivity was underscored in the assertion that many healthcare organisational members may be blind to their own failure to role-model good interpersonal behaviour.

Further reading

O'Neill, O (2002) *A Question of Trust. The BBC Reith Lectures 2002.* New York: Cambridge University Press.

Phillips, A and Taylor, B (2009) *On Kindness.* London: Penguin.

Schön, DA (1987) *Educating the Reflective Practitioner: Toward a new design for teaching and learning in the professions.* San Francisco, CA: Jossey-Bass.

Seddon, J (2008) *Systems Thinking in the Public Sector: The failure of the reform regime . . . and a manifesto for a better way.* Axminster: Triarchy Press.

Concepts and arguments from all of the above books are used in this chapter. Reading them will help you develop your understanding of the inter-related ideas and arguments they contain.

Useful websites

http://www.compassionincare.com

This is the website of Compassion in Care, a charitable movement dedicated to addressing the plight of *victims of silence.* It is interesting to consider the extent to which the existence and activities of this movement are possible because it occupies a critical place outside of public and private healthcare provision, and is thus relatively more free from the constraints of technical rationality and positive public impression management.

https://www.missouriwestern.edu/orgs/polanyi/Duke/Duke2.pdf

This is Polanyi's original lecture outlining his ideas on tacit knowledge. It is hosted on the website of the Polanyi Organization.

https://www.missouriwestern.edu/orgs/polanyi

You may find it interesting to delve into more detail on how Polanyi's ideas were formed and structured into an argument.

http://www.wbuk.org

Whistleblowers UK is a non-profit-making organisation that supports actual and potential whistleblowers from many practice areas, including healthcare.

Glossary

Biomedical model: a model employing the principles of biology, biochemistry, physiology and other basic sciences to solve problems in clinical medicine.

Blip culture: contemporary healthcare cultures where there is only time for brief interpersonal exchanges between nurses and their patients.

Communication: the reciprocal and effective process in which messages are sent and received between two or more people.

Control: is central to good mental health; people who function well at the level of their mental health experience high levels of subjective control; the opposite is true for those who experience mental health difficulties.

Counterculture: the consciously held negative views of a minority of individuals against the dominant culture.

Critical reflexivity: the active practice of personal awareness that goes beyond personal introspection to take into account the social and political contexts and drivers of professional practice.

Cultural relativism: a culture or civilisation where there is the belief that concepts such as right and wrong, goodness and badness, or truth and falsehood are not absolute but change from culture to culture, and situation to situation.

Culture: the dominant mores, habits and beliefs of a group of people, usually united by their ethnic, social, sexual or other orientation.

Culture-centrism: talking, thinking and behaving from a position where one's own culture and cultural identity are assumed to be the 'correct' one, from which other cultures and cultural identities are judged to be lacking, deviant or incorrect.

Discrimination: the conscious or unconscious negative views of individuals, on the basis of their ethnicity, sexual orientation or lifestyle.

Empathy: the ability to be attuned, and respond appropriately, to the inner experience and distress of patients.

Ethnicity: ethnic affiliation or distinctiveness.

Ethnocentricity: the 'taken-for-granted' views held by members of a society, which, they believe, apply globally.

Ethnocentrism: a belief in, or assumption of, the superiority of the social or cultural group that a person belongs to.

Eudaemonistic: basing moral value on the likelihood of actions producing happiness.

Evidence-based practice: the combination of the best available scientific evidence and theories informing safe and effective interpersonal communication in nursing.

Existential-phenomenological: personal experience and responsibility of the individual, who is seen as a free agent, and the doctrine that all knowledge comes from perceptions of what is sensed by the individual.

Experiential learning: learning that is derived from or relating to experience, as opposed to other methods of acquiring knowledge.

Gestalt: a set of things, such as a person's thoughts and experiences, considered as a whole and regarded as amounting to more than the sum of its parts; a set of items or things that are regarded as a whole.

Healthy relating: the use of good communication and interpersonal skills between nurses, their colleagues and their patients; good communication is respectful, non-exploitative, non-judgemental and formal rather than casual.

Helping relationship: a relationship between a nurse and someone in the nurse's care which proves of value to the latter, in regard to helping the person positively move forward in life.

Humanistic approach: implies that individuals can solve their own problems independent of cultural and organisational constraints.

Immigration: coming into a foreign country to settle there.

Individualism: from an 'individualistic' perspective, people are assumed to have the power to find their own solutions to their problems, independent of cultural or organisational constraining factors.

Informatics: the science of processing data for storage and retrieval; information science.

Interpersonal skills: skills that are exhibited when nurses demonstrate their abilities to use evidence-based, and theory-based, styles of communication with their patients and colleagues.

Loss: a feature of the subjective experience of depression or low mood.

Metacognitive: refers to the idea of 'thinking about thinking'; this means, in practice, thinking about the ways in which you, as a nurse, and your patients think about the ways in which you and they think.

Migration: going from one place to another.

Moral practice: in nursing, refers to the respectful treatment of a patient as a fully human being, rather than an object or an 'it'.

Nurse-focused: refers to the defensive ways in which nurses often communicate with their patients; these forms of communication are often guarded, withdrawn and distancing, leaving patients feeling more anxious and lonely than they otherwise might be.

Prejudice: bigoted views held by members of one culture against members of another.

Professional artistry: embodied skilled practice that proceeds from the tacit knowledge resources held by experienced professionals.

Professional friend: a relationship that conforms to the standards of skill, competence or character normally expected of a properly qualified and experienced person in a work environment and combines this with elements of friendship characterised by mutual assistance, approval and support.

Professional relationship: the connection between two or more people or groups and their involvement with one another, especially with regard to the way they behave towards and feel about one another, which is focused around an occupation as a paid job rather than as a hobby.

Rationalisation: finding reasons to explain or justify one's actions.

Reflective writing: writing that is characteristic of and expresses contemplative, analytical and careful thoughts.

Rogerian principles: refers to the position that the 'core conditions' of Rogerian-informed interpersonal communication are both necessary and sufficient; these conditions are 'non-judgementalism', 'unconditional positive regard' and 'genuineness'.

Schemas: psychological templates, or mental structures, that we all develop to make sense of the world; they help us develop general expectations about ourselves, others, social roles and events, and how to behave in specific situations.

Self-awareness: our knowledge about ourselves, our motivations, and how these translate into our behaviours.

Self-esteem: individuals' subjective experience of the overall effectiveness they possess in the conduct of their lives; low self-esteem, therefore, indicates a lowered experience of such effectiveness.

Social relationship: the connection between two or more people or groups and their involvement with one another, especially with regard to the way they behave towards and feel about one another, focused around human society and how it is organised.

Social rules: authoritative principles set forth to guide behaviour or action and that relate to the connection between two or more people or groups and their involvement with one another, especially with regard to the way they behave towards and feel about one another.

Social thinking: use of the mind to form thoughts, opinions, judgements and conclusions about the ways in which people in groups behave and interact.

Suffering: individuals who are suffering exhibit high levels of distress in relation to their physical or mental anguish.

Technical rationality: an approach to practice that matches problems occurring in the professional world with discrete solutions, which arguably takes insufficient account of the complexities of practice.

Theory of mind: the ways in which all human beings make inferences and guesses about what they think is going through the minds of others and what informs their behaviour.

Therapeutic relationship: relates to or involves activities carried out to maintain or improve somebody's health within the professional relationship defined above.

Transcultural: a sophisticated awareness of the beliefs, feelings and behaviours of members of cultures other than one's own.

Unhealthy relating: an abandonment of the moral, psychological and empathic basis for caring, interpersonal communication; organisational environments will contribute to the shaping of healthy and unhealthy relating between nurses and patients.

References

Action on Elder Abuse (2011) *What is Elder Abuse?* Available online at: http://www.elderabuse.org.uk/Mainpages/Abuse/abuse.html (accessed 25 March 2011).

Alvesson, M and Spicer, A (2012) A stupidity-based theory of organizations. *Journal of Management Studies*, 49(7): 1194–1120.

Anderson, N, Calvillo, ER and Fongwa, MN (2007) Community-based approaches to strengthen cultural competency in nursing education. *Journal of Transcultural Nursing*, 18: 49–59.

Aramburu Alegria, C (2011) Transgender identity and health care: implications for psychosocial and physical evaluation. *Journal of the American Academy of Nurse Practitioners*, 23: 175–182.

Armstrong, AE (2006) Towards a strong virtue ethics for nursing practice. *Nursing Philosophy*, 7: 110–124.

Arnold, E and Boggs, KU (2006) *Interpersonal Relationships: Professional communication skills for nurses*, 4th edn. London: Elsevier.

Arnold, E and Boggs, KU (2007) *Interpersonal Relationships: Professional communication skills for nurses*, 5th edn. Philadelphia, PA: WB Saunders.

Arntz, A and Van Gerderen, H (2009) *Schema Therapy for Borderline Personality Disorder.* Chichester: Wiley-Blackwell.

Augoustinos, M, Walker, I and Donaghue, N (2014) *Social Cognition: An integrated introduction*, 3rd edn. London: Sage.

Bach, S (2004) *Psychological Care in Community Nursing: A phenomenological investigation.* PhD thesis, University of Manchester.

Baker, C (2013) Intro. In: Baker, C, Shaw, C and Biley, F (eds) *Our Encounters with Self-Harm.* Ross-on-Wye: PCCS Books.

Baker, C, Shaw, C and Biley, F (eds) (2013) *Our Encounters with Self-Harm.* Ross-on-Wye: PCCS Books.

Balzer-Riley, J (2004) *Communication in Nursing.* Mosby, MO: Mosby/Elsevier.

Banister, P and Kagan, C (1985) The need for research into interpersonal skills. In: Kagan, C (ed.) *Interpersonal Skills in Nursing: Research and applications.* London: Croom Helm, pp44–60.

Baron-Cohen, S (2003) *The Essential Difference: Men, women and the extreme male brain.* London: Basic Books.

Bateson, G (1979) *Mind and Nature.* New York: Dutton.

Baxter, C (2000) Antiracist practice: achieving competency and maintaining professional standards. In: Thompson, T and Mathias, P (eds) *Lyttle's Mental Health and Disorder.* Edinburgh: Bailliere Tindall.

Beck, AT, Rush, AJ, Shaw, BF and Emery, G (1979) *Cognitive Therapy of Depression.* New York: Guilford.

Bendall, E (1976) Learning for reality. *Journal of Advanced Nursing*, 1: 3–9.

Bendall, E (2006) 30th anniversary commentary on Bendall E. 1976 'Learning for reality'. *Journal of Advanced Nursing*, 30th anniversary issue.

Benner, P (1982) From novice to expert. *American Journal of Nursing*, 82(3): 402–407.

Benner, PD (2000) *From Novice to Expert: Excellence and power in clinical nursing practice, commemorative edition.* Upper Saddle River, NJ: Prentice Hall.

References

Benner, P and Wrubel, J (1988) The primacy of caring. *American Journal of Nursing*, 88(8): 1073–1075.

Benner, P, Tanner, C and Chesla, C (1996) *Expertise in Nursing Practice: Caring, clinical judgement, and ethics.* New York: Springer.

Bowlby, J (1988) *A Secure Base: Clinical applications of attachment theory.* London: Routledge.

Broadbent, M, Jarman, H and Berk, M (2002) Improving competence in emergency mental health triage. *Accident & Emergency Nursing*, 10: 155–162.

Brown, B, Crawford, P and Carter, R (2006) *Evidence-based Health Communication.* Maidenhead: Open University Press and McGraw-Hill Education.

Brown, LP (2011) Revisiting our roots: caring in nursing curriculum design. *Nurse Education in Practice*, 11(6): 360–364.

Brykczynska, G (1997) A brief overview of the epistemology of caring. In: Brykczynska, G (ed.) *Caring: The compassion and wisdom of nursing.* London: Arnold/Allen Lane, pp1–9.

Buber, M (1958) *I and Thou*, 2nd edn. New York: Charles Scribner's Sons.

Burnard, P (1996) *Acquiring Interpersonal Skills: A handbook of experiential learning for health professionals*, 2nd edn. London: Chapman and Hall.

Burnard, P (2003) Ordinary chat and therapeutic conversation: phatic communication and mental health nursing. *Journal of Psychiatric and Mental Health Nursing*, 10(6): 678–682.

Burr, V (2003) *Social Constructionism*, 2nd edn. London: Routledge.

Canales, MK (2000) Othering: towards an understanding of difference. *Advances in Nursing Science*, 22: 16–31.

Chant, S, Jenkinson, T, Randle, J and Russell, G (2002) Communication skills: some problems in nursing education and practice. *Journal of Clinical Nursing*, 11: 12–21.

Charlton, CR, Dearing, KS, Berry, JA and Johnson, MJ (2008) Nurse practitioners' communication styles and their impact on patient outcomes: an integrated literature review. *Journal of the American Academy of Nurse Practitioners*, 20: 382–388.

Charon, R (2001) Narrative medicine: a model for empathy, reflection, profession, and trust. *Journal of the American Medical Association*, 286(15): 1897–1902.

Cioffi, J (2006) Culturally diverse patient–nurse interactions on acute care wards. *International Journal of Nursing Practice*, 12(6): 319–325.

Clarke, JB and Wheeler, SJ (1992) A view of the phenomenon of caring in nursing practice. *Journal of Advanced Nursing*, 17: 1283–1290.

Clarke, S, Davies, H, Jenney, M, Glaser, A and Eiser, C (2005) Parental communication and children's behaviour following diagnosis of childhood leukaemia. *Psycho-Oncology*, 14(4): 274–281.

Clay, M and Povey, R (1983) Moral reasoning and the student nurse. *Journal of Advanced Nursing*, 8: 297–302.

Coffield, F, Moseley, D, Hall, E and Ecclestone, K (2004) *Learning Styles and Pedagogy in Post-16 Learning: A systematic and critical review.* London: Learning and Skills Research Centre.

Coleman, J (2011) *The Nature of Adolescence*, 4th edn. London: Routledge.

Cortis, JD (1993) Transcultural nursing: appropriateness for Britain. *Journal of Advances in Health and Nursing Care*, 12(4): 67–77.

Crawford, P (2014) Florence Nightingale carried the lamp but modern nurses carry the can. Available online at: http://theconversation.com/florence-nightingale-carried-the-lamp-but-modern-nurses-carry-the-can-25114 (accessed 9 May 2014).

Davidson, C (1985) The theoretical antecedents to interpersonal skills training. In: Kagan, C (ed.) *Interpersonal Skills in Nursing: Research and applications.* London: Croom Helm, pp22–43.

Davidson, L, Sharp, M and Halford, J (2010) Antisocial and borderline personality disorders. In: Grant, A, Townend, M, Mulhern, R and Short, N (eds) *Cognitive Behavioural Therapy in Mental Health Care,* 2nd edn. London: Sage.

Department for Children, Schools and Families (2004) *The Children Act 2004.* London: Stationery Office.

Department of Health (DH) (2003) *Getting the Right Start: The National Service Framework for Children, Young People and Maternity Services – Standards for Hospitals Services.* London: Stationery Office.

Department of Health (DH) (2004) *Getting Over the Wall: How the NHS is improving the patient's experience.* London: Department of Health.

Department of Health (DH) (2006) *The Expert Patients Programme.* Available online at www.dh.gov.uk (accessed 19 June 2009).

Department of Health (DH) (2010) *Advanced Level Nursing: A position statement.* London: Department of Health.

Department of Health (DH) (2011) *Liberating the NHS: An information revolution: a consultation document.* London: Department of Health.

Department of Health (DH) (2012) *Transforming Care: A national response to Winterbourne View Hospital Department of Health review: final report.* London: Department of Health.

Department of Health (DH) (2013) *Report of the Mid-Staffordshire NHS Foundation Trust Public Inquiry.* London: The Stationery Office.

Devine, F, Savage, M, Crompton, R and Scott, J (eds) (2004) *Rethinking Class: Identities, cultures and lifestyles.* Basingstoke: Palgrave.

DeVito, JA (2007) *The Interpersonal Communication Book,* 11th edn. London: Pearson Education.

Dixon, J and Levine, M (2012) *Beyond Prejudice: Extending the social psychology of conflict, inequality and social change.* Cambridge: Cambridge University Press.

Drury, J (2003) Adolescent communication with adults in authority. *Journal of Language and Social Psychology,* 22(1): 66–73.

Drury, J (2015) The nature of adolescence and its family, societal, community, cultural, and developmental challenges. In: Crome, I and Williams, R (eds) *Substance Misuse and Young People.* London: Hodder & Stoughton (in press).

Drury, J, Catan, L and Dennison, C (1998) Young people's communication difficulties: experiences with employers and family adults. *Journal of Youth Studies,* 1(3): 245–257.

Drury, J, Cocking, C and Reicher, S (2009) Everyone for themselves? A comparative study of crowd solidarity among emergency survivors. *British Journal of Social Psychology,* 48: 487–506.

Economic and Social Data Service (ESDS) (2010) *Annual Population Survey, July 2009–June 2010.* London: ONS.

Edelman, RJ (2000) *The Psychosocial Aspects of the Health Care Process.* Harlow: Prentice Hall.

Egan, EG (1998) *The Skilled Helper: A problem management approach to helping,* 6th edn. Pacific Grove, CA: Brooks Cole.

Erikson, K (2002) Caring science in a new key. *Nursing Science Quarterly,* 15(1): 61–65.

European Union (EU) (2004) *Enabling Good Health for All: A reflection process for a new EU strategy.* Available online at: http://ec.europa.eu/health/ph_overview/Documents/byrne_reflection_en.pdf (accessed 19 June 2009).

Evans, D, Coutsaftiki, D and Fathers, P (2014) *Health Promotion and Public Health for Nursing Students,* 2nd edn. London: Sage Publications.

Falk, JH (2014) Lifelong learning. In: *Encyclopaedia of Science Education*. Netherlands: Springer, pp1–2.

Favretto, AR and Zaltron, F (2013) Children, parents and paediatricians: adequate parenting representations in the therapeutic relation. *Quaderni ACP*, 20: 109–112.

Fennell, M (1999) *Overcoming Low Self-esteem: A self-help guide using cognitive behavioural techniques*. London: Robinson.

Fiske, ST and Taylor, SE (1991) *Social Cognition*, 2nd edn. New York: McGraw-Hill.

Fortman, J (2003) Adolescent language and coomunication from an intergroup perspective. *Journal of Language and Social Psychology*, 22(1): 104–111.

Francis, R (2013) *Report of the Mid Staffordshire NHS Foundation Trust Public Inquiry*. Available online at: http://www.midstaffspublicinquiry.com/report (accessed 4 May 2014).

Freshwater, D and Rolfe, G (2001) Critical reflexivity: a politically and ethically engaged research method for nursing. *NT Research*, 6(1): 526–537.

Frost, PJ, Dutton, JE, Worlen, MC and Wilson, A (2000) Narratives of compassion in organizations. In: Fineman, S (ed.) *Emotion in Organizations*, 2nd edn. London: Sage.

Gerrish, K, Husband, C and Mackenzie, J (1996) *Nursing for a Multi-ethnic Society*. Buckingham: Open University Press.

Gilbert, P (2009) *The Compassionate Mind*. London: Constable.

Gilbert, P and Leahy, R (eds) (2007) *The Therapeutic Relationship in the Cognitive Behavioural Psychotherapies*. Hove: Routledge.

Goffman, E (1959) *The Presentation of Self in Everyday Life*. London: Penguin.

Goffman, E (1972) *Strategic Interaction*. New York: Ballantine.

Goleman, D (2006) *Social Intelligence: The new science of human relationships*. London: Hutchinson.

Grant, A (2000) Clinical supervision and organisational power: a qualitative study. *Mental Health and Learning Disabilities Care*, 31(12): 398–401.

Grant, A (2002) Tales from the order of received wisdom (or some contemporary problems with mental health nurse education in Britain). *Journal of Psychiatric and Mental Health Nursing*, 9: 622–627.

Grant, A (2010a) A brief history of cognitive behavioural therapy. In: Grant, A (ed.) *Cognitive Behavioural Interventions for Mental Health Practitioners*. Exeter: Learning Matters.

Grant, A (2010b) Helping people with borderline personality disorder. In: Grant, A (ed.) *Cognitive Behavioural Interventions for Mental Health Practitioners*. Exeter: Learning Matters.

Grant, A (2010c) Writing the reflexive self: an autoethnography of alcoholism and the impact of psychotherapy culture. *Journal of Psychiatric and Mental Health Nursing*, 17: 577–582.

Grant, A (ed.) (2010d) *Cognitive Behavioural Interventions for Mental Health Practitioners*. Exeter: Learning Matters.

Grant, A (2013) Writing teaching and survival in mental health: a discordant quintet for one. In: Short, NP, Turner, L and Grant, A (eds) *Contemporary British Autoethnography*. Rotterdam: Sense Publishers, pp33–48.

Grant, A (2014a) Breaking the grip: a critical insider account of representational practices in cognitive behavioural psychotherapy and mental health nursing. In: Zeeman, L, Aranda, K and Grant, A (eds) *Queering Health: Critical challenges to normative health and healthcare*. Ross-on-Wye: PCCS Books, pp116–133.

Grant, A (2014b) Neoliberal higher education and nursing scholarship: power, subjectification, threats and resistance. *Nurse Education Today*, 34: 1280–1282.

Grant, A and Townend, M (2007) Some emerging implications for clinical supervision in British mental health nursing. *Journal of Psychiatric and Mental Health Nursing*, 14(6): 609–614.

Grant, A and Leigh-Phippard, H (2014) Troubling the normative mental health recovery project: the silent resistance of a disappearing doctor. In: Zeeman, L, Aranda, K and Grant, A (eds) *Queering Health: Critical challenges to normative health and healthcare.* Ross-on-Wye: PCCS Books, pp100–115.

Grant, A, Mills, J, Mulhern, R and Short, N (2004) *Cognitive Behavioural Therapy in Mental Health Care.* London: Sage.

Grant, A, Townend, M, Mills, J and Cockx, A (2008) *Assessment and Case Formulation in Cognitive Behavioural Therapy.* London: Sage.

Grant, A, Townend, M, Mulhern, R and Short, N (eds) (2010) *Cognitive Behavioural Therapy in Mental Health Care*, 2nd edn. London: Sage.

Grant, A, Biley, F and Walker, H (eds) (2011) *Our Encounters with Madness.* Ross-on-Wye: PCCS Books.

Grant, A, Haire, J, Biley, F and Stone, B (eds) (2013) *Our Encounters with Suicide.* Ross-on-Wye: PCCS Books.

Grant, A, Leigh-Phippard, H and Short, N (2014) Re-storying narrative identity: a dialogical study of mental health recovery and survival. *Journal of Psychiatric and Mental Health Nursing* (in press).

Greenberg, LS (2007) Emotion in the therapeutic relationship in emotion-focused therapy. In: Gilbert, P and Leahy, R (eds) *The Therapeutic Relationship in the Cognitive Behavioural Psychotherapies.* Hove: Routledge.

Greenhalgh, T and Hurwitz, B (1999) Why study narrative. *British Medical Journal*, 318: 48–50.

Grover, SM (2005) Shaping effective communication skills and therapeutic relationships at work: the foundation of collaboration. *American Association of Occupational Health Nurses Journal*, 53: 177.

Hall, ET (1966) *The Hidden Dimension.* New York: Doubleday.

Hallström, I and Runneson, I (2001) Needs of parents of hospitalized children. *Theoria: Journal of Nursing Theory*, 10: 20–27.

Hargie, O (ed.) (2006) *The Handbook of Communication Skills*, 3rd edn. London: Routledge.

Hargie, O and Dickson, D (2004) *Skilled Interpersonal Communication: Research, theory and practice*, 4th edn. London: Routledge.

Hartrick, G (1997) Relational capacity: the foundation for interpersonal nursing practice. *Journal of Advanced Nursing*, 26: 523–528.

Hayes, SC and Smith, S (2005) *Get Out of Your Mind and Into Your Life: The new acceptance and commitment therapy.* Oakland, CA: New Harbinger.

Hebdidge, D (1979) *Subculture: The meaning of style.* London: Routledge.

Henderson, IW (1967) Psychological care of patients with malignant disease. *Applied Therapy*, 9(10): 827–832.

Hendricks, J and Hendricks, CD (1986) *Aging in Mass Society: Myths and realities*, 3rd edn. Boston, MA: Little, Brown.

Henley, A and Schott, J (1999) *Culture, Religion and Patient Care in a Multi-ethnic Society.* London: Age Concern.

Hewitt, JP (1998) *The Myth of Self-esteem: Finding happiness and solving problems in America.* New York: St Martin's Press.

Hofstede, G (1991) *Cultures and Organisation: The software of the mind.* London: McGraw-Hill.

Hogg, MA and Vaughan, GM (2011) *Social Psychology*, 6th edn. Harlow: Pearson Education.

Holstein, JA and Gubrium, JF (2000) *The Self We Live By: Narrative identity in a postmodern world.* New York: Oxford University Press.

Holt, M (2008) The educational preparation of student nurses as communicators of health and wellbeing. *Journal of the Royal Society for the Promotion of Health*, 128(4): 159–160

Honey, P and Mumford, A (1992) *The Manual of Learning Styles.* Maidenhead: Peter Honey.

Howard, A (2001) Fallacies and realities of self. *Counselling and Psychotherapy Journal,* 12(4): 19–23.

Howatson-Jones, L (2013) *Reflective Practice in Nursing,* 2nd edn. London: Sage/Learning Matters.

Howe, D (2013) *Empathy: What it is and why it matters.* Basingstoke: Palgrave Macmillan.

Jasper, M (1996) The first year as a staff nurse: the experiences of a first cohort of Project 2000 nurses. *Journal of Advanced Nursing,* 24: 779–790.

Jones, A (2007) Putting practice into teaching: an exploratory study of nursing undergraduates' interpersonal skills and the effects of using empirical data as a teaching and learning resource. *Journal of Clinical Nursing,* 16: 2297–2307.

Kagan, C, Evans, J and Kay, B (1986) *A Manual of Interpersonal Skills for Nurses: An experiential approach.* London: Harper and Row.

Kitson, AL (2003) A comparative analysis of lay-caring and professional (nursing) caring relationships. *International Journal of Nursing Studies,* 40(5): 503–510.

Kohut, H (1984) *How Does Analysis Cure?* Chicago, IL: University of Chicago Press.

Kolb, DA (2000) *Facilitator's Guide to Learning.* Boston, MA: Hay/McBer.

Kolb, DA and Fry, D (1975) Towards an applied theory of experiential learning. In: Cooper, CL (ed.) *Theories of Group Processes.* Chichester: Wiley.

Kyle, TV (1995) The concept of caring: a review of the literature. *Journal of Advanced Nursing,* 21: 506–514.

Lauder, W, Reynolds, W, Smith, A and Sharkey, S (2002) A comparison of therapeutic commitment, role support, role competency and empathy in three cohorts of nursing students. *Journal of Psychiatric and Mental Health Nursing,* 9: 483–491.

Lea, A, Watson, R and Deary, IJ (1998) Caring in nursing: a multivariate analysis. *Journal of Advanced Nursing,* 28: 662–671.

Leininger, MM (1978) *Transcultural Nursing.* New York: Wiley.

Leininger, MM (1981) The phenomenon of caring: importance, research questions and theoretical considerations. In: Leininger, MM (ed.) *Caring, and Essential Human Need.* Detroit, MI: Wayne State University Press.

Leininger, MM (1984) *Care: The essence of nursing and health.* Detroit, MI: Wayne State University Press.

Leininger, MM (1997) Transcultural nursing research to nursing education and practice: 40 years. *Image: Journal of Nursing Scholarship,* 29(4): 341–347.

Levetown, M (2008) Communicating with children and families: from everyday interactions to skill in conveying distressing information. *American Academy of Pediatrics,* 121(5): 1441–1460.

Levine, M and Crowther, S (2008) The responsive bystander: how social group membership and group size can encourage as well as inhibit bystander intervention. *Journal of Personality and Social Psychology,* 95(6): 1429–1439.

Lewis, CC, Pantell, RH and Sharp, L (1991) Increasing patient knowledge, satisfaction and involvement: randomised trial of a communication intervention. *Pediatrics,* 88(2): 351–358.

Long, A (ed.) (1999) *Interaction for Practice in Community Nursing.* Basingstoke: Macmillan.

Lorig, K, Ritter, P, Dost, A, Plant, K, Laurent, D, and McNeil, I (2008) The expert patients programme online, a 1-year study of an Internet-based self-management programme for people with long-term conditions. *Chronic Illness,* 4(4): 247–256.

Lovering, S (2006) Cultural attitudes and beliefs about pain. *Journal of Transcultural Nursing,* 17(4): 389–395.

Maben, JA, Latter, SB and Clark, JM (2006) The theory–practice gap: impact of professional–bureaucratic work conflict on newly qualified nurses. *Journal of Advanced Nursing,* 55(4): 465–477.

Maben, J, Latter, S and Macleod Clark, J (2007a) The challenges of maintaining ideals and standards in professional practice from a longitudinal study. *Nursing Inquiry*, 14(2): 99–113

Maben, JA, Latter, SB and Clark, JM (2007b) The sustainability of ideals, values and the nursing mandate: evidence from a longitudinal qualitative study. *Nursing Inquiry*, 14: 99–113.

MacLeod Clark, J (1985) The development of research in interpersonal skills. In: Kagan, C (ed.) *Interpersonal Skills in Nursing: Research and applications.* London: Croom Helm, pp9–21.

MacNaught, A (1994) A discriminating service: the socioeconomic and scientific roots of racial discrimination in the National Health Service. *Journal of Inter-Professional Care*, 8: 143–149.

Macpherson of Cluny, W (Chair) (1999) *The Stephen Lawrence Inquiry.* London: Stationery Office.

Maslin-Prothero, S (ed.) (2005) *Bailliere's Study Skills for Nurses and Midwives.* Oxford: Bailliere Tindall.

Maslow, AH (1943) A theory of human motivation. *Psychological Review*, 50(4): 370–396.

McCabe, C (2004) Nurse–patient communication: an exploration of patients' experiences. *Journal of Clinical Nursing*, 13: 41–49.

McCabe, C and Timmins, F (2006) *Communication Skills for Nursing Practice.* London: Palgrave Macmillan.

McCabe, C and Timmins, F (2013) *Communication Skills for Nursing Practice*, 2nd edn. London: Palgrave Macmillan.

McMahon, R (1993) Therapeutic nursing: theory, issues and practice. In: McMahon, R and Pearson, A (eds) *Nursing as Therapy*, 2nd edn. London: Chapman Hall.

Melia, K (1984) Student nurses' construction of occupational socialisation. *Sociology of Health and Illness*, 2(2): 132–151.

Menzies Lyth, I (1988) *Containing Anxiety in Institutions: Selected essays.* London: Free Association Books.

Meyerson, DE (2002) If emotions were honoured: a cultural analysis. In: Fineman, S (ed.) *Emotion in Organizations*, 2nd edn. London: Sage.

Miranda, R and Andersen, SM (2007) The therapeutic relationship: implications from social cognition and transference. In: Gilbert, P and Leahy, RL (eds) *The Therapeutic Relationship in the Cognitive Behavioural Psychotherapies.* Hove: Routledge.

Morgan, G (2006) Organization as psychic prison. In: Morgan, G *Images of Organization*, updated edition. London: Sage Publications.

Morrison, P and Burnard, P (1991) *Caring and Communicating: The interpersonal relationship in nursing.* Basingstoke: Macmillan.

Morse, JM, Bottorff, J, Neander, W and Solberg, S (1991) Comparative analysis of conceptualisations and theories of caring. *Image: Journal of Nursing Scholarship*, 23(2): 119–126.

Morse, JM, Bottorff, J, Anderson, G, O'Brien, B and Solberg, S (1992) Beyond empathy: expanding expressing of caring. *Journal of Advanced Nursing*, 17: 809–821.

Muir Gray, JA (1997) *Evidence-based Healthcare: How to make health policy and management decisions.* New York: Churchill-Livingstone.

Mullen, CA (2005) *Mentorship Primer.* New York: Peter Lang.

Murphy, F, Jones, S, Edwards, M, James, J and Mayer, A (2009) The impact of nurse education on the caring behaviours of nursing students. *Nurse Education Today*, 29(2): 254–264.

Narayanasamy, A (2002) The ACCESS model: a transcultural nursing practice framework. *British Journal of Nursing*, 11(9): 643–650.

Narayanasamy, A and White, E (2005) A review of transcultural nursing. *Nurse Education Today*, 25: 102–111.

National Health Service (NHS) Modernisation Agency (2003) *Essence of Care, Guidance and New Communication Benchmarks.* London: Department of Health.

Newell, R and Gournay, K (eds) (2000) *Mental Health Nursing: An evidence-based approach.* London: Churchill-Livingstone.

Newton, T, Fineman, S and Handy, J (1995) *'Managing' Stress: Emotion and power at work.* London: Sage.

NHS (2009) *Using Mobile Phones in Hospital.* Available online at: http://webarchive.nationalarchives.gov.uk/20130107105354/http:/www.dh.gov.uk/prod_consum_dh/groups/dh_digitalassets/@dh/@en/documents/digitalasset/dh_092812.pdf (accessed 1 September 2014).

NHS England (2014a) *Accessible Information.* Available online at: http://www.england.nhs.uk/ourwork/patients/accessibleinfo-2 (accessed 10 December 2014).

NHS England (2014b) *Patient OnLine.* Available online at: http://www.england.nhs.uk/ourwork/pe/patient-online (accessed 10 December 2014).

Norcross, JC (ed.) (2002) *Psychotherapy Relationships That Work: Therapist contributions and responsiveness to patients.* New York: Oxford University Press.

Nursing and Midwifery Council (NMC) (2004a) *Standards of Proficiency for Pre-registration Nursing Education.* London: NMC.

Nursing and Midwifery Council (NMC) (2004b) *The NMC Code of Professional Conduct: Standards for conduct, performance and ethics.* London: NMC.

Nursing and Midwifery Council (NMC) (2008) *The Code: Standards of conduct, performance and ethics for nurses and midwives.* London: NMC.

Nursing and Midwifery Council (NMC) (2010) *Standards for Pre-registration Nursing Education.* London: NMC.

Nussbaum, JF, Pecchioni, LL, Robinson, JD and Thompson, TL (2000) *Communication and Aging,* 2nd edn. Mahwah, NJ: Lawrence Erlbaum Associates.

Oakes, P, Haslam, A and Turner, J (1994) *Stereotypes and Social Reality.* Oxford: Blackwell.

Oliver, M (1990) *The Politics of Disablement.* London: Macmillan.

O'Neill, O (2002) *A Question of Trust: The BBC Reith Lectures 2002.* New York: Cambridge University Press.

Ousey, K and Johnson, M (2007) Being a real nurse – concepts of caring and culture in the clinical areas. *Nurse Education in Practice,* 7(3): 150–155.

Padesky, C (1991) Schema as self-prejudice. Reprinted from the *International Cognitive Therapy Newsletter,* 6: 6–7 (1990).

Parfitt, B (1998) *Working Across Culture: A study of expatriate nurses working in developing countries in primary health care.* Aldershot: Ashage.

Peel, N (2003) Critical care: the role of the critical care nurse in the delivery of bad news. *British Journal of Nursing,* 12: 966–971.

Perrin, EC, Lewkowicz, C and Young, MH (2000) Shared vision: concordance among fathers, mothers, and paediatricians about unmet needs of children with chronic health conditions. *Pediatrics,* 105: 277–285.

Petrie, P (1997) *Communicating with Children and Adults: Interpersonal skills for early years and play work.* London: Arnold.

Pfeffer, J (1981) *Power in Organizations.* Marshfield, MA: Pitman Publishing.

Phillips, A and Taylor, B (2009) *On Kindness.* London: Penguin.

Plato (344c) (2004) *Plato's Republic.* Indianapolis: Hackett.

Platt, L (2005) *Migration and Social Mobility: The life chances of Britain's minority ethnic communities.* London: Joseph Rowntree Foundation.

Polanyi, M (1967) *The Tacit Dimension.* New York: Doubleday.

Prilleltensky, I, Nelson, G and Peirson, L (2001) The role of power and control in children's lives: an ecological analysis of pathways towards wellness, resilience and problems. *Journal of Community and Applied Social Psychology,* 11(2): 143–158.

Prosser, J (2013) Judith Butler: queer feminism, transgender, and the transubstantiation of sex. In: Hall, DE, Jagose, A, with Bebell, A and Potter, S (eds) *The Routledge Queer Studies Reader.* London and New York: Routledge.

Quinn, F and Hughes, S (2007) *Quinn's Principles and Practice of Nurse Education.* Oxford: Nelson Thornes.

Radsma, J (1994) Caring and nursing: a dilemma. *Journal of Advanced Nursing,* 20: 444–449.

Rapley, M, Moncrieff, J and Dillon, J (eds) (2011) *De-Medicalizing Misery: Psychiatry, psychology and the human condition.* Basingstoke: Palgrave Macmillan.

Reed, S and Standing, M (2011) *Successful Professional Portfolios for Nursing Students.* Exeter: Learning Matters.

Rees, C and Sheard, C (2004) Undergraduate medical students' views about a reflective portfolio assessment of their communication skills learning. *Medical Education,* 38: 125–128.

Reynolds, WJ and Scott, B (2000) Do nurses and other professional helpers normally display much empathy? Integrative literature reviews and meta-analyses. *Journal of Advanced Nursing,* 31(1): 226–234.

Richardson, L (1997) *Fields of Play (Constructing an Academic Life).* New Brunswick, NJ: Rutgers University Press.

Riley, AW (2004) Evidence that school-aged children can self-report on their health. *Ambulatory Pediatrics,* 4 (Suppl. 4): 371–376.

Robb, M and Douglas, J (2004) Managing diversity. *Nursing Management UK,* 11(1): 25–29.

Rodgers, BL and Cowles, KV (1997) A conceptual foundation for human suffering in nursing care and research. *Journal of Advanced Nursing,* 25: 1048–1053.

Rogers, CR (1961) *On Becoming a Person.* Boston, MA: Houghton Mifflin.

Rogers, CR (1967) *On Becoming a Person: A therapist's view of psychotherapy.* London: Constable.

Rogers, CR (2002) *Client Centred Therapy.* London: Constable.

Rose, D and Pevalin, DJ (2005) *The National Statistics Socio-economic Classification: Origins, development and use.* Institute for Social and Economic Research, University of Essex. Basingstoke: Palgrave Macmillan.

Ruesch, J (1961) *Therapeutic Communication.* Toronto: Norton.

Ryan, EB and Hamilton, JM (1994) Patronizing the old: how do younger and older adults respond to baby talk in the nursing home? *International Journal of Aging and Human Development,* 39(1): 21–32.

Sackett, D, Strauss, S, Richardson, W and Haynes, R (2004) *Evidence Based Medicine: How to practise and teach EBM.* London: Churchill Livingstone.

Sapir, E (1983) In: Mandelbaum, DG (ed.) *Selected Writings of Edward Sapir in Language, Culture and Personality.* Berkeley, CA: University of California Press.

Sawley, L (2001) Perceptions of racism in the Health Service. *Nursing Standard,* 15(19): 33–35.

Schön, D (1987) *Educating the Reflective Practitioner: Toward a new design for teaching and learning in the professions.* San Francisco, CA: Jossey-Bass.

Seddon, J (2008) *Systems Thinking in the Public Sector: The failure of the reform regime . . . and a manifesto for a better way.* Axminster: Triarchy Press.

Shields, L, Morrall, P, Goodman, B, Purcell, C and Watson, R (2012) Care to be a nurse? Reflections on a radio broadcast and its ramifications for nursing today. *Nurse Education Today*, 32: 614–617.

Siviter, B and Stevens, D (2004) *The Student Nurse Handbook: A survival guide.* Oxford: Bailliere Tindall.

Sloane, J (1993) Offences and defences against patients: a psychoanalytical view of the borderline between empathic failure and malpractice. *Canadian Journal of Psychology*, 38: 265–273.

Smail, D (2011) Psychotherapy: illusion with no future? In: Rapley, M, Moncrieff, J and Dillon, J (eds) *De-Medicalizing Misery: Psychiatry, psychology and the human condition.* Basingstoke: Palgrave Macmillan, pp226–238.

Smircich, L (1983) Concepts of culture and organizational analysis. *Administrative Science Quarterly*, 28: 339–358.

Smith, A (1997) Learning about reflection. *Journal of Advanced Nursing*, 28: 891–898.

Smith, A and Jack, K (2005) Reflective practice: a meaningful task for students. *Nursing Standard*, 19: 33–37.

Smith, CE (1987) *Patient Education: Nurses in partnership with other health professionals.* Orlando, FL: Grune & Stratton.

Smith, S and Grant, A (2014) Facial affect recognition and mental health. *Mental Health Practice*, 17(10): 12–16.

Speed, E (2011) Discourses of acceptance and resistance: speaking out about psychiatry. In: Rapley, M, Moncrieff, J and Dillon, J (eds) *De-Medicalizing Misery: Psychiatry, psychology and the human condition.* Basingstoke: Palgrave Macmillan, pp123–140.

Spichiger, E, Walhagen, MI and Benner, P (2005) Nursing as a caring practice. *Scandinavian Journal of Caring Science*, 19: 303–309.

Stanley, JC, Hayes, J, Fredrick, L and Silverman, R (2014) Examining student nurses' perceptions of diverse populations: are student nurses prepared to care for culturally diverse patients? *Journal of Nurse Education and Practice*, 4(7): 148–155.

Sternberg, RJ (2001) *In Search of the Human Mind*, 3rd edn. Fort Worth, TX: Harcourt College.

Stokes, G (1991) A transcultural nurse is about. *Senior Nurse*, 11(1): 40–42.

Tait, A (1985) Interpersonal skill issues arising from mastectomy contexts. In: Kagan, C (ed.) *Interpersonal Skills in Nursing: Research and applications.* London: Croom-Helm, pp165–184.

Tajfel, H (ed.) (1982) *Social Identity Intergroup Relations.* Cambridge: Cambridge University Press, pp15–40.

Tates, K and Meeuwesen, L (2001). Doctor–parent–child communication: a review of the literature. *Social Science and Medicine*, 52: 839–851.

Taylor, S, Leigh-Phippard, H and Grant, A (2014) Writing for recovery: a practice development project for mental health service users, carers and survivors. *International Practice Development Journal*, 4(1): 1–13.

Teekman, B (2000) Exploring reflective practice in nursing. *Journal of Advanced Nursing*, 31: 1125–1135.

Theodosius, C (2008) *Emotional Labour in Health Care: The unmanaged heart of nursing.* London: Routledge.

Thompson, D (ed.) (1995) *The Concise Oxford Dictionary of Current English*, 9th edn. Oxford: Clarendon Press.

Thompson, N (2001) *Anti-discriminatory Practice*, 3rd edn. Basingstoke: Palgrave Macmillan.

Thurlow, C (2005) Deconstructing adolescent communication. In: Williams, A and Thurlow, C (eds) *Talking Adolescence: Perspectives on communication in the teenage years.* New York: Peter Lang.

Thwaites, R and Bennett-Levy, J (2007) Conceptualizing empathy in cognitive behaviour therapy: making the implicit explicit. *Behavioural and Cognitive Psychotherapy*, 35: 591–612.

Timmins, F (2007) Communication skills: revisiting the fundamentals. *Nurse Prescribing*, 5: 395–399.

Toffler, A (1980) *The Third Wave.* New York: William Morrow.

Trinder, L and Reynolds, S (eds) (2000) *Evidence-based Practice: A critical appraisal.* Oxford: Blackwell.

Turner, JC, Hogg, MA, Oakes, PJ, Reicher, SD and Weatherell, MS (1987) *Rediscovering the Social Group: A social categorisation theory.* Oxford: Blackwell.

United Nations (1989) *United Nations Convention on the Rights of the Child.* Geneva: United Nations.

Walthew, P and Scott, H (2012) Concepts of health promotion held by pre-registration nurses in four schools of nursing in New Zealand. *Nurse Education Today,* 32(3): 224–228.

Watson, J (1988) *Nursing: Human science and human care,* 3rd edn. New York: National League for Nursing.

Watson, J (1997) The theory of human caring: Retrospective and prospective. *Nursing Science Quarterly,* 10(1): 49–52.

Watson, J and Foster, R (2003) The attending nurse caring model: integrating theory, evidence and advanced caring-healing therapeutics for transforming professional practice. *Journal of Clinical Nursing,* 12(3): 360–365.

Whitton, E (2003) *Humanistic Approach to Psychotherapy.* Chichester: Wiley Blackwell.

Whorf, B (1956) In: Carroll, J (ed.) *Language, Thought and Reality: Selected writings of Benjamin Lee Whorf.* Boston, MA: MIT Press.

Wilkins, H (1993) Transcultural nursing: a selective review of the literature, 1985–1991. *Journal of Advanced Nursing,* 18: 602–616.

Williams, A and Garrett, P (2005) Intergroup perspectives on ageing and intergenerational communication. In: Harwood, J and Giles, H (eds) *Intergroup Communiction: Multiple perspectives.* New York: Peter Lang, pp93–115.

World Health Organization (WHO) (2000a) *World Health Report 2000 – Health Systems: Improving performance.* Geneva: WHO.

World Health Organization (WHO) (2000b) *Nurses and Midwives for Health: A WHO strategy for nursing and midwifery education.* Copenhagen: WHO Regional Office for Europe.

Wrate, RM (1992) Talking to adolescents. In: Myerscough, PR (ed.) *Talking with Patients: A basic clinical skill,* 2nd edn. Oxford, UK: Oxford University Press.

Wurzbach, ME (1999) The moral metaphors of nursing. *Journal of Advanced Nursing,* 30(1): 94–99.

Wyer, RS and Srull, TK (1986) Human cognition in its social context. *Psychological Review,* 93: 322–359.

Young, R, Sweeting, H and West, P (2006) Prevalence of deliberate self harm and attempted suicide within contemporary Goth youth subculture: longitudinal cohort study. *British Medical Journal,* 332(7549): 1058–1061.

Zeeman, L, Aranda, K and Grant, A (2014a) Queer challenges to evidence-based practice. *Nursing Inquiry,* 21(2): 101–111.

Zeeman, L, Aranda, K and Grant, A (eds) (2014b) *Queering Health: Critical challenges to normative health and healthcare.* Ross-on-Wye: PCCS Books.

Zimbardo, P (2009) *The Lucifer Effect.* London: Rider.

Index

Note: References in **bold** are to the glossary; those to tables and figures are indicated as '13*t*' '14*f*.'